OXFORD MEDICAL PUBLICATIONS

Disablement in the Community

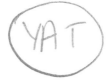

Disablement in the Community

EDITED BY

DONALD L. PATRICK

AND

HEDLEY PEACH

OXFORD NEW YORK TORONTO MELBOURNE
OXFORD UNIVERSITY PRESS
1989

Oxford University Press, Walton Street, Oxford OX2 6DP
Oxford New York Toronto
Delhi Bombay Calcutta Madras Karachi
Petaling Jaya Singapore Hong Kong Tokyo
Nairobi Dar es Salaam Cape Town
Melbourne Auckland
and associated companies in
Berlin Ibadan

Oxford is a trade mark of Oxford University Press

Published in the United States
by Oxford University Press, New York

British Library Cataloguing in Publication Data
Disablement in the community.
1. Great Britain. Handicapped persons.
Community care
I. Patrick, Donald L. II. Peach, Hedley
362.4'0458'0941
ISBN 0–19–261434–7

Library of Congress Cataloging in Publication Data
Disablement in the community / edited by Donald L. Patrick and Hedley
Peach.
p. cm.—(Oxford medical publications)
Includes bibliographies and index.
1. Community health services. 2. Chronically ill—Care. 3. Home
care services. I. Patrick, Donald L. II. Peach, Hedley.
III. Series.
[DNLM: 1. Disability Evaluation. 2. Handicapped. 3. Home Care
Services. 4. Rehabilitation. WB 320 D6105]
RA425.D54 1989   (362.1'0425–dc19)   (DNLM/DLC)   88–25379
ISBN 0–19–261434–7 (pbk.)

Typeset by Cambrian Typesetters, Frimley, Surrey
Printed in Great Britain by
Biddles Ltd.
Guildford and King's Lynn

Preface

It is now widely accepted that the balance of health and social care for people with disability should shift from being institutional or residential to care in the community. This change in policy is based on the assumption that disabled people can and do enjoy a higher quality of life living in their own homes and surrounded by those families and friends who are willing and able to give them the needed support. Few would argue with this objective of community care for those disabled people who need and desire it. To implement a community care policy, however, requires information that has been missing until now. Most previous work has concentrated on handicapped children, registered disabled people, or elderly people in or about to enter institutions. This book is among those helping to develop community care policy by focusing on disabled adults aged 16–75 living in their own homes.

A complete picture of the burden of chronic illness on the life of this section of the community demands a socio–medical definition of disablement. Knowledge of the relative importance of medical conditions and social support in determining the level of disability in the community and how this varies over time is also essential. Identifying health and social service policies to enhance the quality of life of disabled people living in the community requires rigorous appraisal of the alternative strategies for providing financial and formal service support. This volume shows how knowledge of the epidemiology of disablement can help planners, service providers, and voluntary organizations choose strategies for community care.

A study of the full consequences of disease, in terms of impairment, disability, and handicap, requires a broad perspective on the medical causes of disability and their social implications. The first chapter of the book discusses how the disabilities and handicaps associated with various types of physical, intellectual, and psychological impairments, vary widely in their nature and course. A broad definition of disablement, including medical conditions and their consequences for social and economic activities, provided the basis for a survey to identify disabled residents in the community as described in Chapter 2. Fifteen per cent of the adults living in an inner-city area reported disability, but only 5 per cent of these people had injuries, defects, or other physical problems. The traditional image of disability is thereby challenged by the large number of people who reported that some health problem was restricting their lives in a way which was important to them.

How to measure the severity of disability when so broadly defined is a complex problem discussed in Chapter 3. An instrument called the Functional Limitations Profile (FLP) has been devised to assess the many areas of everyday life in which disabled people are affected. The varying functional limitations and activity restrictions have been combined into more global or summary indices which are also useful in evaluative studies and clinical trials with disabled populations. The use of the self-care measure of disability, which has been recommended for local government surveys of disability in Britain, is compared with the FLP. The self-care measure failed to identify some individuals reporting significant psychosocial and physical disability on the FLP. These disabled people would be overlooked if the self-care measure were the sole basis for identifying need for services.

The pattern of disability over time is described in Chapter 4. Nearly a quarter of all disabled people report that their disability steadily deteriorates over time, while another quarter steadily improve, a quarter report no significant changes, and the last quarter show a highly variable pattern.

Chapter 5 describes how a significant amount of disability in the community can be accounted for by only a small number of impairments. Some of these impairments are associated with social disability alone, and their burden on the community can and has been underestimated by instruments which assess only the physical dimension of disability. Most of the symptoms associated with disability have, in fact, been reported to doctors and are being treated. Moreover, people who have not reported the few untreated disabling symptoms tend to be the less severely disabled. Paradoxically the treatment of symptoms and medical conditions can also lead to disability; the role of commonly prescribed drugs in the aetiology of disability is examined in Chapter 6.

The development of community care for disabled people

involves a large number of different health and social provisions, both in terms of the services provided by formal and informal carers and financial support given to disabled people by the government. The social and political rationale for allocation in cash or kind differ. Chapter 7 tackles the assumptions and the problems involved in defining and measuring the need for community care and in formulating health and social policies which emphasize cash benefits or services. These problems are confounded when considering a universal benefit or service for all disabled people in the community, many of whom are disabled, but not severely so, and mainly in the psychosocial areas of their lives. Similarly, Chapter 8 discusses the economic issues involved in constructing a fair and workable incomes and employment policy for all disabled people.

Family members, relatives, friends, and neighbours not only form important sources of practical assistance and care, but also provide psychosocial support to disabled people. Such support has been shown to act as a protective factor in relation to the onset and course of illness. Chapter 9 examines the availability of support both from individual network members and through participation in social groups and organizations. The characteristics of people with low levels of psychosocial support are described, and the consequences of a lack of support on the course of disability is considered.

While previous chapters have been concerned with impairment and disability, Chapter 10 deals with the nature and determinants of handicap or disadvantage. The problems that disabled people encounter in everyday life and their own efforts at solving or containing them are described using qualitative interview data from men and women who suffer from rheumatoid arthritis.

Broadening the definition of disability increases the number of people in the community who are counted as 'disabled' people and about whom health and personal social services need to be concerned. In Chapter 11, information about the factors associated with the course of disability and about the services they currently use is discussed in the context of planning a strategy for community care. Primary prevention efforts need to be targeted, particularly at strokes, if the level of disability in the community is to be reduced significantly. There is limited scope for reducing the level of disability in the community through increasing the general practitioner's or family doctor's awareness and treatment of impairment through screening for unreported medical complaints among the disabled. There is scope, however, for reducing the iatrogenic component of disability.

A large number of social contacts in some way protects disabled people from a decline in their functioning. Expecting formal services to substitute for a lay network or trying to provide the kind of support normally provided by relatives and friends through self-help groups, however, presents a number of difficulties. The disabled with a large number of social contacts tend to be employed, and increasing employment opportunities for the disabled may be the most practical way of providing appropriate and effective support. The relative lack of comparative need for formal services in a broadly defined sample of disabled people does not support a policy to increase provision of these services. Disabled people, however, do need help, especially in coping with handicap. Although many disabled people use their own resources to cope with disadvantage, the strategies they employ sometimes result in social isolation. Devising and providing services to meet *every* need of the disabled person is not feasible. The only viable alternative is to make compensatory provision for the handicap in cash. It is with this issue that further research and debate on disablement policy should be concerned.

Each chapter of this book applies research findings from the Lambeth disablement studies to planning or policy questions concerned with community care for disabled people. Neither the studies nor the findings cover each question completely, and pertinent literature is reviewed and cited where additional support or evidence for a finding, or method, or a point of view is needed. A considerable amount of time has elapsed since the completion of these studies and the appearance of this volume. The major issues addressed and the investigative approaches are nevertheless relevant to the contemporary discussion of disability policy and research.

Translating data into information or policy recommendations involves a subtle blend of critical thought, solid data, insight in interpretation, and forceful presentation of a conclusion or a perspective. The contribution of each individual investigator has been presented with the overall objective of suggesting what should be considered in formulating policy and what disablement policy should be pursued. Many different perspectives are involved in such policy formulation, including the clients and their families, administrators, professionals, and policy advocates. The multi-disciplinary team of authors represented in this book brings many of these different perspectives to bear on the issues that concern people in the community.

The reader of this book may be one of the myriad of people concerned with the planning and provision of care of those living with chronic illness in their homes, whatever the nature of that illness or its severity. Much of the information currently available on disablement in the community has been collected from people with specific conditions at different points in time. This makes a community approach to the planning of interventions very difficult. Although one diagnosis of the problems in a single urban area cannot answer all the complex research and policy questions, the problems will be similar regardless of the community and its location. We hope that our socio–medical approach to the detection of disability and to mapping the course of disability over time in a single community will help planners, service providers, and voluntary organizations adopt a more cohesive and compre-hensive approach to the community care of disabled people.

1988   D. L. P.
                                                               H. P.

Acknowledgements

The Lambeth studies of disablement represent the multi-disciplinary efforts of a great number of people over an 8-year period. While the authors are now located across the globe, the studies were planned in 1977 by the Project Team on the Health and Care of the Physically Disabled in Lambeth under the direction of Donald Patrick at St. Thomas's Hospital Medical School in London. David Locker, Stephen Green, Sarah Darby, Geoffrey Horton, Andrew Creese, and Cathy Taylor helped design the overall strategy of the investigation. The postal screening and community survey methodologies were tested in 1977 at a general practice at Kingston-on-Thames where Michael D'Souza and Ian Gregg provided access to patients. Cathy Taylor co-ordinated the intensive fieldwork to screen 10 per cent of Lambeth households to identify disabled residents. Dick Wiggins and Yoga Sittampalam joined the team to help in the analysis of the prevalence data and in preparing the community survey sample. Headly Peach assumed the role of medical adviser, participating in the Lambeth Health Survey and taking over local responsibility for the study in 1983–84. John Charlton, Myfanwy Morgan, Ellie Scrivens, Sheena Somerville, David Locker, and Peter West all took responsibility for major areas of the survey. Ruth Silver, Barbara Caufield and Nicholas Simms helped in the analysis of survey data. Under the direction of Jane Ritchie and Jean Morton-Williams, staff of Social and Community Planning Research carried out the innumerable tasks of survey fieldwork for the longitudinal study. Sheena Somerville and Yoga Sittampalam took major responsibility for the value scaling study to provide severity weights for the measure of disability used in the survey with assistance from Peter Sweetnam and Angus Rodgers. David Locker conducted the qualitative study of handicap and its determinants. Ellie Scrivens planned and conducted the study of priorities for resource allocation in cash or in kind, with the assistance of Barbara Caufield. Particular thanks go to Johannes Goldschmidt, David

Clyde, and George Iwaniak for seeing the project through the computer at St. Thomas's and the University of London.

Walter Holland has provided support and advice from the very beginning of this investigation, having been closely involved in the earlier Lambeth health studies in the 1960s. His continuous encouragement to a changing, multi-disciplinary research team made it possible to mount a long-term programme of research. Other colleagues have given us important direction and advice at different times, in particular, Jean Weddell and David Morrell. Juliana Oladuti helped to administer the Project and its component studies.

Many people were involved in the preparation of this manuscript. We would like to thank particularly Katherine Smart, who copy-edited most of the chapters in collaboration with the senior editor. Thanks also go to V. Norcott Martin, of the Medical Illustration Department at the Rayne Institute, St. Thomas's Hospital for producing the illustrations used in this book from the contributors' rough sketches. Kathy Cheek and Lorene Neubauer worked with Donald Patrick to produce the final manuscript for the publishers.

All the studies reported in this volume were supported financially by the Department of Health and Social Security. Additional support was provided during the initial stages by the Special Trustees of St. Thomas's Hospital. We are very grateful for this support and for the guidance provided by Jeremy Metters and Doreen Rothman, our principle DHSS liaison offiers, as well as the individual members of the Physically Handicapped Research Liaison Group.

Scientific and practical advice and criticism from many different sources outside St. Thomas's helped to shape each study from the beginning. We are particularly indebted to Margot Jeffreys, Philip Wood, Michael Warren, and the late Amelia Harris for their help in planning the investigation. Leonard Syme, Ann Cartwright, Karen Dunnell, Marilyn Bergner, Bill Carter, Ted Bennett, Derek Duckworth, Richard Stowell, Bruce Clifford, and Shirley Beresford gave important advice along the way. At the same time, we acknowledge the inevitable errors, both recognized and unrecognized, as our own.

The residents of Lambeth have given us their time and their support in all studies reported here. We are encouraged by how much they care about disabled people and what should be done for them. Each participant deserves our thanks for their contribution to the development of social and health policy for disablement in the years ahead.

The material in chapters 4, 5, and 6 was originally published in the Journal of Epidemiology and Community Health and is reproduced here with the kind permission of the editor and publishers.

Contents

Contributors

Donald L. Patrick PhD., MSPH
Department of Health Services,
University of Washington,
Seattle, Washington USA.

Hedley Peach, BSc, MB, BCh, PhD., MFCM
Tropical Health Surveillance Unit,
James Cook University of North Queensland,
Queensland, Australia.

John R. H. Charlton, BSc, MSc
Department of Health and Social Security,
London, England.

David Locker, BDS, PhD
Faculty of Dentistry,
University of Toronto,
Toronto, Canada.

Myfanwy Morgan, BA, MA
Department of Community Medicine,
United Medical and Dental Schools,
St. Thomas's Hospital,
London, England.

Ellie Scrivens, PhD
Institute of Public Sector Management,
London Business School,
London, England.

Peter West, PhD
Touche Ross Management Consultants,
Hill House,
1, Little New Street,
London EC4A 3TR

1

A socio–medical approach to disablement

DONALD L. PATRICK

Each disease has in many instances been denoted by three or four terms, and each term has been applied to as many different diseases; vague, inconvenient names have been employed or complications have been registered instead of primary diseases. The nomenclature is of as much importance in this department of enquiry as weights and measures in the physical sciences and should be settled without delay.

William Farr, *First Annual Report of the Registrar General*,
London, 1839

Disablement is a major social problem. It affects not only the people who are disabled, but also their families and friends, their health and social care providers, and all members of their communities. In a contemporary welfare state, disablement is a major pathway to public aid. Many different institutions treat disabled people or provide them with housing and other provisions, including schools, hospitals, and community organizations. Disabled people themselves sometimes organize into active interest groups within a community. Furthermore, the stigmatizing effects of disablement often reach beyond disabled people, bringing disadvantage to their families and friends as well. Thus, disablement touches every member of society at one level or another.

Disablement does not affect everyone in the same way, however, mainly because the abilities, interests, resources, and social activities of disabled people are just as varied as those of healthy individuals. People with medical conditions as diverse as arthritis, chronic bronchitis, or spinal injury, for example, require different kinds of help at different times in their lives, depending on such factors as age, education, family support, and their immediate physical and social environment. Even people with the same medical conditions will experience differences in the stability, improvement, or deterioration of their conditions. On the other hand, disabled people have much in common. All too often they share the disadvantages of restricted mobility, loss of income, lack of work opportunity, prejudice, or lack of independence, despite clear differences in the nature and course of their conditions.

Such variations in the medical, psychological, and social conditions of disabled people, coupled with their need for equal opportunities, demands a move away from the traditional disease-oriented approach to disablement, which tends to disregard the importance of social and psychological factors. The disease-oriented approach focusses on the biomedical with medical care as the primary service provision, the physician as expert, and the patient in a 'sick role' of dependency. We need, instead, a socio–medical approach that incorporates both the medical and the social perspectives in assessing, preventing, and caring for people with disabling conditions.

The socio–medical approach augments the strictly medical knowledge about any disability by also examining the communities where the people live, their work opportunities, and their families. The large number of services required to meet specific needs are considered in light of the circumstances in which chronically ill people and their families live. Controversial issues of social policy towards disabled people, such as mobility allowances, income supplements, or special employment provisions, are seen in relation to their effects on the community as a whole, and on disabled people's sense of membership in that community, rather than in terms of their direct effects upon the disabled alone.

Throughout the world, policy-makers and analysts, epidemiologists, various service professionals, and other groups who help disabled people, have recognized the need for a broad socio–medical perspective on disablement. Nagi (1969) noted that equitable decisions about the qualifications of disabled applicants and clients in a democratic, pluralistic society require universally-accepted criteria and terminology. He observed that terms such as 'pathology', 'impairment', 'functional limitation', and 'disability' were used in various ways by different programmes, and that these variations influenced the provision of services and benefits. Nagi concluded that the notion of 'limitation in function' provided a useful supplement to an assessment based on pathology or impairment alone. However, the broader social context, such as a changing labour market or the decreased prestige of, and value placed on, older people, also affects society's perception and treatment of disabled people. The employability and perceived attractiveness of people with stable and unalterable limitations is influenced by the economy and culture in which they live. Thus, the concept of a broad continuum of disability must be accepted if we are to reflect both common characteristics and individual needs. This continuum can be used by various decision-makers in delivering services, in assessing needs, in allocating resources, and in planning for community provision.

The concept of disablement

A continuum of disability has been proposed by the World Health Organization (1980) in terms of a classification of impairments, disabilities, and handicaps that might be used in conjunction with the widely applied International Classification of Diseases (ICD). This proposed classification is based on the work of Wood and his colleagues at the University of Manchester in the UK (Wood 1975, 1980; Wood and Badley 1980). Developed over the last decade, the WHO classification system defined:

(1) *Impairment* as any loss or abnormality of psychological, or physiological, or anatomical structure or function;
(2) *Disability* as any restriction or lack (resulting from an impairment) of ability to perform an activity in the manner or within the range considered normal for a human being;
(3) *Handicap* as a disadvantage for a given individual, resulting from impairment or a disability, that limits or prevents the fulfillment of a role that is normal (depending on age, sex, and social and cultural factors) for that individual.

Disablement is a collective term referring to any experience that is a consequence of disease and which may be identified as impairment, disability, or handicap. The use and utility of these disablement terms will be assessed during the Tenth Revision Conference of the International Classification of Disease in the early 1990s. Although the definitions were developed to help classify disablement, the scheme also has potential for either assessing disabled individuals in surveys or determining eligibility for benefits, pensions, or other income provisions.

In the World Health Organization scheme the interrelationship among disablement concepts is depicted as a linear progression from the disease or disorder to functional limitations (impairment), restrictions in activity (disability), and social disadvantage (handicap). Disorders of function, including the systems of mental function, are considered impairments. In an earlier version of the scheme, functional limitations were classified as disabilities (Wood 1975). Because the boundary between impairment and disability seemed unclear, functional limitations in the final trial classification were considered impairments.

In our view, the boundary between functional limitations and activity restrictions is unclear, particularly for psychological processes such as disturbances in emotions, affect, and mood that may involve, for example, 'anxiety', 'depression', or 'irritability'. The distinction is also unclear for the impairment of drives such as 'decrease of libido' or 'impairment of heterosexual role' (World Health Organization 1980, pp. 62–3). Such limitations in function often are deviations from a socially-defined norm or standard for behaviour, not intrinsic characteristics of individuals nor organic disturbances. Thus, in our view some of these functional limitations are better defined as disabilities that may or may not cause disadvantage. Deviation from normative behaviour may also be viewed as a disadvantage where stigma results without a functional limitation or activity restriction.

Interrelationships among the three disablement concepts are depicted in Fig. 1.1. The most important feature of this scheme is the hypothesized progression from the intrinsic situation and organ level to social consequences. Impairment is seen as becoming evident in an individual's physical circumstances, first through functional limitations and then through activity restrictions. In this case, the progression can be altered or incomplete depending on the nature of the impairment, the internal and external environment of the individual, and the social definition of the situation. The scheme also indicates that the state of handicap is defined by different groups in society, and that these groups may have varying values about what is usual or expected in terms of behaviour and social conditions. For example, people with limited

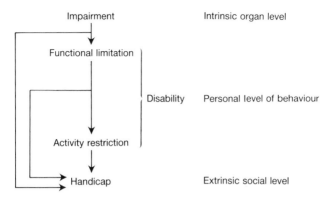

Fig. 1.1. Interrelationships among disease consequences.

mobility may find it difficult to drive a car or to use public transportation. How disadvantageous this is will depend upon the individual's age, work role, family support, availability of special transportation, and so on.

The conceptual scheme shown in Fig. 1.1 also indicates the various sequences or relationships among the experiences of impairment, disability, and handicap. Handicap may result from impairment without a major restriction in activity, as in the case of a facial disfigurement. Similarly, one can be disabled without necessarily being handicapped, depending on the goals and resources of the disabled person. Individuals with the same level of impairment also may differ considerably in how disabled or handicapped they are, depending on their attitudes and their social and cultural situations. Having a hurt finger, for example, may not prevent many people from pursuing normal activities, but it could be devastating to a professional piano player. It is also important to note that impairments and disabilities may be visible or invisible, temporary or permanent, and progressive or regressive (World Health Organization 1981).

The scheme shown in Fig. 1.1 has important implications for the assessment of individuals and populations with disablement, the provision of preventive and treatment services, and the formulation of social policy. Chapters 2 and 3 deal with the identification and assessment of disabled persons. Subsequent chapters take up the implications of impairment, disability, and handicap for service provision and policy formulation. Before these questions are considered, however, it is important to consider how the concepts of impairment, disability, and handicap fit into the public health or community context of prevention and planning for health and social policy.

Primary, secondary, and tertiary prevention

To establish a framework for identifying the preventive aspects of chronic disease, the US Commission on Chronic Illness (1949–56) proposed the classification of disease prevention into two major types—primary and secondary (Commission on Chronic Illness 1957). Primary prevention refers to practices or measures that are taken prior to the start of the disease to avert the occurrence of the chronic condition. An example would be averting chronic obstructive pulmonary disease by reducing smoking among the population. Secondary prevention, which begins after the disease is recognized, is dedicated to 'halting the progression of a disease from its early unrecognized stage to a more severe one and preventing complications or sequelae of disease' (Commission on Chronic Illness 1957, p. 16). Although not defined here in precise terms, 'sequelae of disease' may include disability, recurrent episodes of illness, and/ or suffering. Secondary prevention usually refers to case-finding or screening for symptoms of disease and to the immediate actions taken during examination and diagnosis, for example, prescribing betablockers for individuals with significantly elevated blood-pressure. However, because chronic illness is long-term and progressive, such dynamic aspects of prevention were regarded as tertiary prevention in later discussions of chronic disease. Tertiary prevention usually consists of continuing measures designed to prevent progression or deterioration in the disease condition, such as exercise therapy for patients with chronic obstructive lung disease.

Primary prevention has been subdivided further to distinguish between primordial preventive measures taken before risk factors are present and strictly primary measures taken to eliminate risk factors. For example, educational campaigns before people begin smoking, or breath analysis of drivers for alcohol before automobile accidents happen, constitute primordial prevention. On the other hand, smoking cessation classes or toxic waste clean-up are examples of primary preventive measures.

The distinction between primary and secondary prevention depends on the identification of the biological origins of disease. The concept of biological origin is becoming progressively more diffuse as more is learned about multifactorial chronic diseases. There may be periods during which the underlying disease process is present before the clinical illness is apparent. For example, myocardial infarction can be viewed as starting with the first arterial wall lesions rather than with the first chest pains. Similarly, abnormal increases in blood-sugar, blood-pressure, or serum cholesterol may not produce discomfort or disability, although each may have serious prognostic importance for future clinical events.

In the conceptual scheme of disablement, viewed as planes of experience by Wood and Badley (1980), deviation from the norm may or may not be recognized at the same time that impairment occurs. Impairments do not have to be linked to specific aetiology, and the 'definition of what constitutes impairment is undertaken primarily by those qualified to judge physical and mental functioning, according to generally accepted standards'. Thus, primary prevention of impairment must refer to all measures aimed at reducing the occurrence of impairments, visible or invisible. These measures include all of the traditional public health activities regarding the environment, vaccination, health education, improvement of nutrition, control of harmful substances, reduction of accidents, elimination of occupational hazards, and other cultural, social, and environmental programmes.

Once a person or a professional has detected pathology, with or without symptoms, the major thrust is secondary prevention, or the limiting or reversing of disability caused by impairment. Recognition of the disease may occur at the level of disability and may involve functional limitations (considered as impairments in the WHO scheme) or restrictions of activity that may make the affected person seek professional advice. Secondary prevention activities include early detection and treatment, reduction in risk factors, vocational and educational counselling, and social interventions.

Tertiary prevention of disablement refers to measures designed to prevent the disability from becoming handicap. These measures may be directed towards the person, his or her immediate

environment, or society as a whole. Some definitions of 'rehabilitation' are similar to those of tertiary prevention in terms of
providing therapy that may reduce disadvantage, but tertiary
activities also encompass broader social-policy initiatives. Such
efforts include compensation and access legislation as well as self-
help initiatives, all of which lead to the removal of physical, social,
political, and economic barriers, and to the full participation of
disabled people in society. Those measures may help reverse
disability as well as increase independence and promote social
integration. For many permanently disabled people, tertiary
prevention is the main way to safeguard their rights and to reduce
the distance between society and themselves.

As noted by the World Health Organization (1981), disability
prevention differs significantly in developed and developing
countries. The major causes of disabling impairments in developing
countries are malnutrition, communicable disease, low-quality
perinatal care, and accidents. In developed countries most
disabilities are caused by accidents (especially among the younger
population); chronic somatic diseases such as rheumatic disorders
and cardiovascular, pulmonary, and psychiatric illness; genetically-
induced impairments; chronic pain and injuries; and chronic
alcohol, smoking, and drug abuse. Paradoxically, modern medical
technology and therapeutic measures may increase the incidence
of disability by allowing patients with severe disabling conditions
to survive longer. This book is concerned mainly with disablement
in developed countries, where the major causes of disability are
chronic disease processes.

At the level of primary prevention, community-based provision
is unlikely to exist for people who experience impairment,
disability, or handicap. This situation is true, even though disease
prevention and health promotion may well avert the occurrence of
some impairments and disabilities, particularly those related to
ischaemic heart disease, accidents, or specific occupational risks
(Office of the Assistant Secretary for Health 1979, 1980). Yet the
dominance of social and behavioural risk-factors such as smoking,
obesity, and stress, which are among the leading causes of
disablement, suggests that primary prevention strategies are not
enough to eliminate disablement.

Secondary prevention measures such as screening and health
examinations can help in the early detection and treatment of

disabling conditions, including hypertension, diabetes, and hearing or sight loss (Canadian Task Force on the Periodic Health Examinations 1979). Multifactorial screening of entire middle-aged populations, however, has proved ineffective and expensive (South-East London Screening Study Group 1977).

Public health policy is often concerned, and rightly so, with primary prevention at the society, community, and individual level. However, the effects of primary prevention on disease incidence and severity emerge only gradually over the decades, especially when lifestyle changes are involved. Social provision for chronic disease has to be based mainly on disability and handicap, where the major concerns are to limit restrictions on activity and to reduce or eliminate any associated disadvantages. Furthermore, the failures of primary prevention are likely to be with us for the indefinite future.

As the proportion of the population that is older increases, there is a growing emphasis on chronic disease and disablement. With more people living longer, common chronic conditions have emerged as major causes of death and disability. A longer life expectancy may well be accompanied by a rising incidence of chronic diseases among older people. These diseases are common but seldom fatal, such as arthritis and other musculoskeletal disorders (Verbrugge 1984). This aging of the population is a worldwide phenomenon among industrialized nations (Rice and Feldman 1983). Thus second- and third-level prevention activities will become more and more important.

The primary concern in this book is with community measures that will use and enhance local, regional, and national resources. These measures are directed at reducing the impact of disabling and handicapping conditions and enabling disabled and handicapped people to achieve social integration. The behavioural consequences and social experience of disablement motivate efforts to plan community services, to legislate, to provide benefits, and to establish public policy at all levels for persons with disabilities and handicaps.

The Lambeth studies of disablement

The theoretical scheme suggested by the WHO classification provided a broad socio–medical perspective for investigating disablement among adults living at home in the London Borough of Lambeth. Conducted between 1977 and 1983, the Lambeth studies represent an effort to apply a socio–medical approach to the gathering of information for social policy development and for strategic planning decisions concerning physically disabled people living in the urban community.

The investigation involved five interrelated studies:

(1) a screening study to identify a sample of disabled persons and to estimate the prevalence of disability among those living at home in the Borough of Lambeth;
(2) a longitudinal disability interview survey (Lambeth Health Survey) conducted in three phases over 2 years to investigate the individual, social, and environmental factors associated with physical disability;
(3) a value scaling study to measure the perceived severity of dysfunction associated with functional limitations and activity restrictions;
(4) a study of the social and economic consequences of disability to develop a better understanding of handicap and how it is influenced by social situations;
(5) a priorities study to examine the preference for cash benefits or local authority services among disabled people, relatives, and friends who care for them, and planners and providers of services.

These five studies were intended to provide a better understanding of the health status and variety of needs experienced by physically impaired, disabled, and handicapped people. A multimethod, multi-stage research strategy was needed to investigate the wide diversity of impairments consequent to disease and equally varied social circumstances and service demands of disabled people.

No single investigation is likely to capture the complexity of the relationship between disablement and the community. For example, the removal of architectural barriers, the improvement of educational opportunities, the provision of disability income maintenance, and the development of self-help organizations are all important and central issues to any discussion of public policy and disablement. While these issues were important concerns of respondents in the Lambeth studies, they were not the single focus of attention. The Lambeth studies were planned as a community enquiry to provide information on the epidemiology of disablement in that community and to apply the information to health and social policy questions affecting that community, and disabled people in general.

Studies of the distribution and determinants of disablement in populations are relatively new to the field of epidemiology. Solutions to the problems of disabled people and the design for intervention strategies, as well as their implementation, are likely to emerge only after investigation and debate within and across communities. Experience in collecting and applying epidemiological data is necessary to shape effective, efficient, and equitable policy for disabled people in their respective communities. The Lambeth studies represent extensive experience with an inner city area and contribute to this emerging research and planning model.

Assessment of community needs

The use of epidemiological methods and data for policy formulation in the field of disablement means assessing population needs, either implicitly in the measures of health status or explicitly in the interpretation of results. The determination of 'need' for planning and programming is a complicated matter. The information required for planning community provision is different from that required to assess the needs of individuals for immediate help, since principles of fairness and rationing are involved. These principles are discussed more fully in Chapter 7 in relation to the allocation of resources. Before presenting epidemiological findings on impairment, however, the concept of 'need' requires explanation.

Bradshaw (1972) has distinguished four categories of need:

(1) felt need can be described as that perceived by the individual in terms of want;
(2) expressed need corresponds roughly to economic demand, since only some felt needs are expressed;
(3) normative need refers to the way an expert, usually a professional, defines need in a given situation;
(4) comparative need is the principle on which 'territorial justice'

is based, i.e. if X and Y have similar characteristics and Y receives a service or benefit not received by X, then X is considered to be in need.

While this taxonomy does not resolve all the difficulties in assessing need in epidemiological surveys, it does offer a framework for interpreting the results of community surveys of health status or disability. Self-reports of functional limitations, activity restrictions, or service needs clearly do not constitute normative need. And while many professionals may agree on the absolute needs for individuals in terms of nutrition, physical activity, or safety, there is less agreement about what constitutes adequate housing or even adequate emotional functioning. Furthermore, poor health status cannot in itself be regarded as a need for service provision. The availability of an effective means of influencing a particular health state should be considered, for example, in the determination of what is preventable mortality or morbidity (Rutstein *et al.* 1976). The availability of resources is also relevant.

Most self-reported information on health, service use, social support, and so on, which is collected in surveys, concerns felt or expressed needs. When people with similar levels of disability are compared in terms of the amount of support they receive from family or public sources, we are dealing with comparative need. Information on felt, expressed, or comparative need cannot give a clear picture of the *unmet* needs in a community, since policy and priorities determine whether provisions can be made to meet a particular need.

Survey information can indicate the lack of expressed, felt, or comparative need. Reliable and valid reports of such need can help planners assess how well their priorities for services match expressions of need. Planners also should be aware of how the current distribution of resources is evaluated by those who benefit and those who do not. Such information is critical to the continuing process of planning the content of services and benefits, and in deciding who should receive help.

Community and the Borough of Lambeth

The Borough of Lambeth is defined by its geographical boundaries rather than by the functions or activities of the people living within its boundaries. Some writers distinguish between various levels of community, starting with the family or household as the smallest unit and aggregating outwards to neighbourhood, county (or local authority), region, nation, and finally humanity as a whole. Geographical boundaries sometimes imply mutual inter-dependence among groups of people, if only that those who live and work within the boundaries interact with each other more than they do with people outside these boundaries.

Applying the term 'community' to an inner city area such as Lambeth can lead to confusion if a strict 'functional' definition is suggested. Areas of cities clearly are not orderly arrangements of functions and interdependencies. The multitude of neighbour-hoods, organizations, formal or informal associations, parishes, and other groups criss-cross and overlap to such an extent in modern urban areas that one might ask 'where is the community?'

Lambeth is better described as a set of diverse 'communities', ranging from the relatively affluent neighbourhoods near the South Bank complex to the Brixton area that has been the site of racial strife and riots. These areas or neighbourhoods do not conform to a single community type or divide into an artificial characterization of communities. Rather, they are locally-based networks that may be defined by ethnic origin, type of housing, history of residence, shopping district, or some other social or cultural determinant of interaction. People in these areas constitute a community to the degree that they share a sense of common identity.

In this book, community refers not only to groups of people sharing a common identity, but also, in a broader sense, to any non-institutional household where people live with family and/or friends. A community thus consists of persons in social interaction within a geographic area and having one or more additional common tie (Hillery 1955). Disabled people living in the 'com-munity' in an urban area have patterns of social ties that are influenced by the ethnic groups and types of social networks to which they belong (see Chapter 9). In this case both definitions of community—a sense of common identity and a household or residence—overlap. Both are important when we discuss the health and social needs of disabled people.

A third definition of community is employed when we consider a borough-wide policy for community care of disabled people. All residents of Lambeth comprise the community when considering physical disability and public policy. Equal or unequal opportunity, non-discrimination or reverse discrimination, integration or segregation, free choice, and access are key issues that involve all residents of a defined area of political organization. The entire 'community' has to be involved if disabled people are to realize their rights as citizens.

A map of the Borough of Lambeth is shown in Fig. 1.2. The local authority area consists of 2,727 hectares divided into 20 electoral wards. In 1975, Lambeth was shown to be one of 20 Scottish, Welsh, and English authorities with large numbers of people experiencing the worst housing and unemployment problems in the three countries (Department of Environment 1975). Additional powers have been granted to the local authority of Lambeth to arrest and reverse its problems, and legislation exists to help strengthen the local economy (London Borough of Lambeth 1982). The problems of disabled people in Lambeth are inextricably linked to the wider social and economic problems of the area. Developing resources for disabled residents and using them effectively will undoubtedly be influenced by the structure and dynamics of the borough.

The population of Lambeth reached a peak of 421,000 in 1931 and since then has continuously declined by about 1.4 per cent a year during the 1970s and early 1980s. Approximately 244,143 people were counted as residents during the 1981 census (Office of Population Censuses and Surveys 1982). Just under one in four of the borough's population were born outside the UK with nearly the same proportion living in households where the head was born in the New Commonwealth or Pakistan. There are relatively fewer households with children than in England, but 20 per cent of these children are in one-parent families.

The number of jobs in the borough has been declining by about 2 per cent a year and an estimated 21 per cent of its residents between the ages of 16 and 64 (59 for women) who have been in the labour market are out of employment. Half the borough's jobs are in central and local government, the health services, and public utilities. Thirty per cent of the households contain one person living alone, with 15 per cent being one pensioner living independently. Nearly half of the households in Lambeth are now rented, from the two main housing authorities or a housing

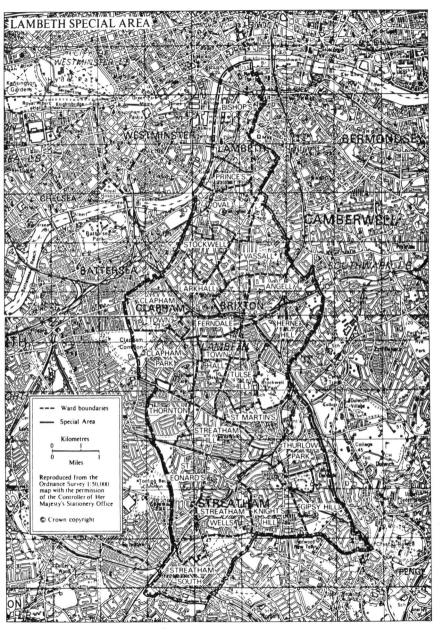

Fig. 1.2. Map of the London Borough of Lambeth.

association. Nine per cent of the households lack or share the use of a bath, and almost 60 per cent do not have a car. The most common type of dwelling is the purpose-built, high- and low-rise flat, constructed as part of an extensive rehousing programme carried out in the 1960s.

Lambeth has received much attention from legislators, policy-makers, and researchers. Much of this attention has focused on the problems of immigrant populations and the housing, employment, crime prevention, social, and health needs shared by all areas of urban deprivation. Lambeth's infant mortality is among the highest in London, and major efforts are being made to improve the early identification of mothers and infants at risk and to develop intensive follow-up programmes. While the standardized mortality ratio for Lambeth is close to the national average (101:100), there has been little information up until now on the type and incidence of illness suffered by local residents.

The Lambeth disablement studies were undertaken to investigate the problems of physical illness and disability experienced by residents of the borough. While estimates of the prevalence of mental or emotional disorder were obtained (see Chapter 2), the main survey was limited to people with physical impairments. People with mental or emotional disorders were not excluded because they were thought to be unimportant to the health and social services or because they did not have acute social needs, but because separate planning and research bodies existed in the borough for mental handicap and mental illness. Those who were impaired solely in vision or in hearing also were not included in the interview studies. Likewise, their needs are the concern of separate research and service departments in the nation as a whole. Since the information gap concerned the other general classes of disability in adults, the Lambeth studies were designed to investigate those needs and to suggest a strategy for community provision.

References

Bradshaw, J. (1972). A taxonomy of social need. In *Problems and progress in medical care: essays on current research* (ed. G McLachlan). Oxford University Press, Oxford.
Canadian Task Force on the Periodic Health Examinations (1979).

Periodic health examination. *Canadian Medical Journal* **121**, 1193–1254.

Commission on Chronic Illness (1957). *Chronic illness in the United States*, Vol 1. Harvard University Press, Cambridge, Massachusetts, USA.

Department of the Environment (1975). *Census indicators of urban deprivation: working note number 6*. Department of the Environment, London.

Hillery, G. A. (1955). Definitions of community: areas of agreement. *Rural Sociology* 20(a): 111–25.

London Borough of Lambeth (1982). *A Guide to the Lambeth Inner City Partnerships*. Lambeth Borough, London.

Office of the Assistant Secretary for Health (1979). *Healthy people: Surgeon General's report on health promotion and disease prevention* Government Printing Office, July, Stock no. 017–001–004160–2 Washington, DC, USA.

Office of the Assistant Secretary for Health (1980). *Promoting health, preventing disease: objective for the nation*. Government Printing Office, Stock No. 017–001–00435–9; Washington, DC, USA.

Office of Population Censuses and Surveys (1982). *Greater London Supplement–2: Lambeth Special Area*. OPCs County Monitor, Reference CEN 81 CM 17/S2. OPCS, London.

Rutstein, D., Berenberg, W., Chalmers, T., Child, C., Fishman, A., and Perrin, E. (1976). Measuring the quality of medical care clinical method. *New England Journal of Medicine* **294**, 582–3.

Nagi, S. Z. (1969). *Disability and rehabilitation: legal, clinical and self-concepts and measurement*. Ohio State University Press Columbus, Ohio, USA.

Rice, D. P. and Feldman, J. J. (1983). Living longer in the United States: demographic changes and health needs of the elderly. *Health and Society* **61**, 362–96.

South-East London Screening Study Group (1977). A controlled trial of multiphasic screening in middle age: results of the South-East London Screening Study. *International Journal of Epidemiology* **6**, 356–63.

Verbrugge, L. (1984). Longer life but worsening health? *Health and Society* **62**, 475–519.

Wood, P. H. N. (1975). *Classification of impairments and handicaps* (WHO/ICD9/REF. Conf/75.5). World Health Organization, Geneva.

Wood, P. H. N. (1980). The language of disablement: a glossary relating to disease and its consequences. *International Rehabilitation Medicine*, **2**, 86–92.

Wood, P. H. N. and Badley, E. M. (1980). *People with disabilities: towards acquiring information which reflects more sensitively their problems and needs*. World Rehabilitation Fund, Washington, DC, USA.

World Health Organization (WHO) (1980). *International classification of impairments, disabilities and handicaps*. WHO, Geneva.

World Health Organization (WHO) (1981). *Disability prevention and rehabilitation*. Technical Report Series 66B. WHO, Geneva.

2

Screening for disability

DONALD L. PATRICK

It shall be the duty of every local authority having functions
under Section 29 of the National Assistance Act 1948 to
inform themselves of the number of persons to whom that
section applied within their area and of the need for the
asking by the authority of arrangements under that Section
for such persons.

Chronically Sick and Disabled Persons Act, 1970, UK

Finding out how many disabled people live in a community and
what their problems and needs are is not a straightforward task.
Although planners and professionals have access to three important information sources, the data from these sources do not always
portray the extent of disablement accurately. To use this information
intelligently, anyone planning disablement policy needs to understand the various strengths and weaknesses of each data source.

The initial information often comes from estimates of the
prevalence of disablement calculated from national surveys. These
surveys have been conducted frequently, sometimes on a continuing basis, to provide information about the number of
disability days, functional incapacities, or work limitations in a
defined population, usually among adults aged 16 and above. The
second source of routinely available data is local registers and
service records of people with medical conditions, different types
of disabilities and handicaps, or specific health and social service
needs. The third source is *ad hoc* studies of patients who seek care
from health and social services.

Unfortunately, estimates of disability prevalence obtained from
national surveys often fail to reflect the particular social and
economic conditions of a local community. They make assumptions
about the geographical distribution of important characteristics
such as age, sex, and ethnic origin that may not be valid for a
particular community. Likewise, data taken from different surveys

or statistical bases are highly prone to variations in quality, sensitivity, and specificity. Individuals with multiple impairments, for example, may be counted more than once. Furthermore, simple measures of disability days do not distinguish between the effects of acute illness, which are characterized by severe but short-term incapacity, and chronic illnesses, which present a possible progression of symptoms and intermittent exacerbations that are sometimes heightened by additional acute illnesses. While the distinction between acute and chronic disability may not have a significant influence on estimates of current resource requirements, making projections of service needs for chronically disabled people requires less ambiguous data.

Estimating the prevalence of disablement is not the same as identifying all the disabled and handicapped people in a community. Sampling of a population for interview obviously misses some disabled persons (OPCS, 1983). The only alternative is a complete population survey. The total population survey strategy has been applied successfully in studies in the city of Canterbury, England (Warren 1974; 1983), and in various surveys in the UK conducted by Outset, a disablement information unit (Agerholm 1975). The Canterbury studies reached 96 per cent of all households in the community while the Outset studies, using volunteer interviewers, collected questionnaires from approximately 75 per cent of the populations studied. Neither set of studies included people living in institutions such as hospitals, homes for the elderly, or nursing homes. The World Health Organization has supported total population surveys in developing countries to obtain estimates of the prevalence of impairing conditions, including those surveys that account for persons residing in institutions (World Health Organization 1981).

Most communities, however, cannot afford the cost of conducting a total population survey, so strategies for designing and implementing sample surveys in the community have been developed in England (Harris and Head 1974). Similarly, the Health Interview Survey, which was conducted with a sample of the US population, provides annual estimates of disability on a national basis (National Center for Health Statistics 1981).

Registers and service records of various categories of impaired and disabled people, such as people with multiple sclerosis, cerebral palsy, or other crippling diseases, also are readily available. These records may be kept by official health and social service authorities or by voluntary agencies. Registration is usually voluntary, although official registers may render persons eligible for services or cash benefits. In some cases disability information is contained in categorical disease registers, such as cancer or tumour registers, which provide epidemiological information on particular populations. Not all disabled people are aware of disease, disability, or handicap registers, however, and some disabled people do not wish to be on any register. Surveys in England have shown repeatedly that many disabled people eligible for social service benefits and services are not on statutory registers maintained by the local authorities. The Canterbury studies demonstrated that registers and records do not identify all handicapped people in a community. While registers and records may be used in management and planning, their main use is for the individual care of clients or patients.

Patients with disabling diseases such as multiple sclerosis, rheumatoid arthritis, or chronic obstructive pulmonary disease sometimes are interviewed in *ad hoc* studies, which are designed to describe the natural history of a condition, estimate its incidence, or evaluate intervention strategies. These studies usually involve medical examinations or the collection of clinical data to determine medical case needs or to evaluate the success of a preventive strategy (Jeffreys *et al.* 1969). Studies of patients can, of course, be biased by selection, in that those who seek care often differ significantly from those who do not, whether in severity of condition, attitude, compliance with recommended treatment, or the many social and psychological characteristics important to prevention or management. Problems of defining 'who is a case' may also plague such studies, particularly if the criteria are wide and open to disagreement, as in studies of mental illness in the community (Wing *et al.* 1981).

Estimates of prevalence

Regardless of the methods used for identifying disabled persons—household surveys, local registers, or patient studies—British estimates of the prevalence of disablement in the community vary widely, according to the definition and measures of impairment, disability, or handicap used, and the assumptions made in calculating population estimates. Most population studies have been carried out in two stages: postal identification, followed by interview. Some surveys have assumed that non-respondents are not disabled. Not all of the interviewers have been trained, and in some local surveys, the questionnaires and interview schedules contained questions that had not been tested for repeatability and validity (Knight and Warren 1978). These and other variations in survey design have resulted in a history of conflicting and incomparable estimates.

In 1968, Bennett and his colleagues (1970) conducted a two-stage, postal and interviewer follow-up prevalence survey of disability among people aged 15 and over living in north Lambeth in London. The authors reported prevalence estimates of 6.5 per cent for men and 8.1 per cent for women. At the same time, the Office of Population Censuses and Surveys (OPCS) administrated a two-stage survey on a substantial national sample (Harris 1971). The OPCS National Survey estimated there were more than 3 million impaired people aged 16 or over living in private households in Great Britain, many of whom had difficulty coping with normal daily activities and were often isolated, practically housebound, unknown to any official agency, and receiving little if any assistance. People were defined as impaired 'if they lacked all or part of a limb or had a defective organ or mechanism of the body'. Those of them who had difficulty in carrying out one or more self-care activities were defined as 'handicapped'. These impaired people constituted 3.9 per cent of the population aged 16–64 and 27.8 per cent of the population aged 65 and over (Buckle 1971).

Thirty seven per cent of the impaired in the OPCS National Survey were estimated to be severely or appreciably handicapped, according to a set of criteria concerned with self-care: getting to or using the toilet, feeding, doing up buttons and zippers, getting in and out of bed, having a bath or all-over wash, washing hands and face, putting on shoes and socks or stockings, dressing, combing and brushing hair, or shaving. The numbers of impaired and handicapped people increased strikingly among the older age groups. Disability of appreciable or more severe degree was encountered almost twice as frequently in women as in men, the rates being 36.9 and 19.5 per 1,000 adults, respectively. Marked regional differences were noted in the prevalence of impairment with higher rates in the south-west of Britain and lower rates in the south-west.

This model government survey focused attention on the need for services for disabled people. The sheer weight of the numbers of handicapped indicated the potential advantage in helping families cope with their disabled members for as long as possible. As a result of this study, the major aim of services for the physically disabled became the provision of appropriate support services and care within the community.

Following the OPCS National Survey, many local authorities in Great Britain conducted similar prevalence studies to implement the 1970 Chronically Sick and Disabled Persons Act (Knight and Warren 1978). The Act was designed to compel local authorities to seek out impaired people in their area, and, where necessary, to provide them with domestic help, home nursing, holidays, and recreational activities. Where community care was impossible to provide, residential care was to be offered. These survey studies have estimated that 4–8 per cent of the population are physically impaired, and that of these, a third to a half are handicapped or experience significant disadvantage from their impairments (Knight and Warren 1978).

Nothing like the OPCS National Survey had ever been done before, and it remains the most comprehensive source of statistics on disability in adults in Britain, although a new national survey with a focus on eligibility for disability benefits is underway. Using these and other national data on mental handicap, mental illness, and sensory loss, Wood and Badley (1978) have estimated that 34.3 per cent of adults in Great Britain have some kind of impairment. Refraction errors are the most common problem, followed by mental illness and non-traumatically acquired physical impairments. Among these impaired adults, one-tenth or 3.5 per cent are estimated to be severely disabled with impairments that interfere significantly with functional performance and activity.

In the USA, the Health Interview Survey annually selects a sample of about 40,000 households, representing approximately 120,000 persons. One respondent from each household is interviewed extensively to ascertain the state of health of each resident, including any functional limitations attributable to a chronic health condition. Recent survey results estimated that 14.4 per cent of the non-institutionalized population in the US was limited in activities by a chronic health condition (National Center for Health Statistics 1985). An estimated 10.9 per cent are considered more severely disabled, such that they cannot carry on their major activities of working, keeping house, or engaging in school or pre-school activites. The estimated rates have remained essentially level in the period 1978–81 after a short term in which the rates appeared to be increasing (Colvez and Blanchet 1981). The most plausible reasons for the increased reports of disability in this continuing survey were: a heightened awareness of health in the population due to earlier diagnosis; lower death rates; and more empathetic and flexible public attitudes about disability. While procedures for the National Health Interview Survey questionnaire and data collection have changed in several significant ways, there is no evidence that these changes have affected observed trends in self-reported disability (Wilson and Drury 1984). The proportion of the population for which some limitation was reported increased with age, from 3.8 per cent for those under age 17 to 45.7 per cent for those over 65.

The US National Health Interview Survey also has provided estimates of the need for assistance in everyday activities in the community (National Center for Health Statistics 1983). The proportion of adults requiring functional assistance increased with age, particularly for those needing help with bathing, dressing, eating, using the toilet, getting in and out of bed or a chair, or taking care of a device to control bowel movements or urination. Two per cent of adults aged 65–74 required such help compared with 18 per cent of those aged 85 and over.

The Survey of Income and Education, conducted in 1974 by the US National Health Interview Survey of the Census, provided more detailed statistics on 158,500 households, where disablement was defined as having a chronic health condition that prevented participation in a major activity appropriate to one's age group (US Bureau of the Census 1979). This survey indicated that 17.6 per cent of the black population were disabled, compared with 13.7 per cent of the white population. People classified as Hispanic were found to have the lowest rate of disability: 10.6 per cent. The prevalence of disability rose significantly with increasing age and with lower levels of education and income. Prevalence also varied by as much as 45 per cent from one region of the country to another, with New England having the lowest rate (12.6 per cent) and the south-east region the highest (18.3 per cent).

The two major sources of US data just cited indicate that similar estimates are obtained (14–17 per cent) when disability is defined as having a chronic condition that prevents participation in a major activity appropriate for age, such as school, work, or housework. Surveys by the OPCS and local authorities in Britain suggest that consistently lower estimates (4–8 per cent) are derived using more narrow criteria related to ambulation, mobility, and self-care items. Another difference between British and US data is that the US estimates are calculated from large-scale household interview surveys administered at considerable cost, while the British estimates come from national and local studies that were conducted using a variety of data-collection methods and interviewers.

In addition to considering the technical and cost aspects of survey design and procedures, any community group studying the distribution of disablement has to decide on a definition of disability, a method for identifying and sampling disabled respondents, and a strategy for estimating prevalence and the need for health and social services from the sample survey data. The 1978 Lambeth screening study illustrates the significance of these decisions on study results. It also provides an example of the benefits and limits of prevalence data for local planning of health and social services. For a review of the more technical aspects of disability surveys, see Harris and Head (1974) or Duckworth (1984).

The Lambeth screening study

The aim of the 1978 Lambeth screening study was to estimate the prevalence of impairment and disabilities in the population living at home and to develop a model of the factors most strongly associated with disability. The study is an example of a low-cost, one-stage, postal strategy for identifying disabled persons most likely to require services or benefits. The results help identify the relative contributions of a disability definition to the prevalence estimate, an important piece of information for communities attempting to design local identification and prevalence surveys.

A postal questionnaire was developed in the Lambeth study to screen for disability in private households (Peach *et al.* 1980;

Patrick *et al.* 1981, 1982). (Appendix I contains a copy of the questionnaire). The questionnaire consisted of 25 screening items, a section on illness conditions causing disability, and household information. The disability screening items fell into four broad categories:

1. Ambulation and mobility—walking, negotiating stairs, going outside the house, crossing the road, travelling on a bus or train.
2. Body care and movement—getting in and out of bed or a chair, dressing, kneeling or bending, bathing, holding or gripping, controlling bowels or bladder, toileting.
3. Sensory and motor—giddiness or fits, frequent falls, weakness or paralysis of extremities, stroke, visual difficulties, hearing difficulties, loss of extremity.
4. Social activity—illness-related limitations in working, doing the job of choice, doing housework, visiting family or friends, or engaging in other social activities.

Respondents were asked to describe the major illnesses or disabling conditions for any household member reported to have a functional limitation or an activity restriction. They also were asked basic household information, including the sex, year of birth, marital status, and current employment status of each member. Because of the possible adverse effects on response rate, ethnic origin was not recorded on the postal questionnaire.

Respondents were classified as disabled if they met established criteria for a significant activity restriction or functional limitation and if they reported the underlying medical condition or impairment associated with the restriction or limitation. Included in the criteria were difficulties with one or more of (1) the ambulation, mobility, body care, or movement items, *except* constipation or stress incontinence alone; (2) the sensory–motor items; and/or (3) the social activity items, *except* limitation in working or doing the job of choice where the respondent was over retirement age. Medical conditions were coded using the International Classification of Diseases (8th Revision).

Ten per cent of private households listed on the local electoral register were sampled, and the relative chance of the household appearing in the sample was used in calculating prevalence estimates. The response rate after an initial mailing, two reminders, and personal follow-up was 87 per cent. Visits to a 10 per cent sample of addresses that gave no response indicated that most of them were unoccupied households.

The estimated prevalence of disability in Lambeth households by age and sex is shown in Table 2.1. It is estimated that 17.9 per

Table 2.1. *Estimated prevalence of disabled persons aged 16 or over living at home in Lambeth by age and sex*

Age groups (years)	Estimated per cent † and (numbers) ‡					
	Males		Females		All persons	
16	3.0	(1 000)	3.4	(1 100)	3.2	(2 100)
30–49	6.1	(2 100)	8.6	(2 900)	7.4	(5 000)
50–64	17.9	(4 200)	18.2	(4 700)	18.1	(8 900)
65–74	27.2	(2 900)	32.4	(4 500)	30.1	(7 400)
≥ 75	43.3	(1 800)	60.6	(5 700)	55.1	(7 500)
All ages	12.5	(12 000)	17.9	(18 900)	15.4†	(30 900)

†Standard error of estimate = 0.18.
‡Estimates for 1977 rounded to the nearest hundred using GLC population projection figures for Lambeth.

cent of women and 12.5 per cent of men had some functional limitation or activity restriction. Overall, 15.4 per cent of the population aged 16 and above was estimated to be disabled. The validity of studies using postal surveys may be affected by non-responders, since such surveys require more co-operation on the part of the respondent. Thus there is a greater chance that responders and non-responders will differ. Late reponders to the survey tended to be less disabled than early responders. Allowing for possible non-responder bias, the prevalence estimate reduced from 15.4 per cent to 14.8 per cent (Locker *et al.* 1981). The prevalence of disability increased with age for both sexes, and women consistently reported disability more frequently than men

Screening for disability

for all age groups and item categories. The most frequently reported functional limitations were hearing difficulties (4.5 per cent), weakness and paralysis (3.3 per cent), and difficulty seeing newspaper print, even with eyeglasses (3.9 per cent). Difficulty with housework was the most frequently reported social activity restriction.

Fig. 2.1 shows the major disabling conditions reported by men

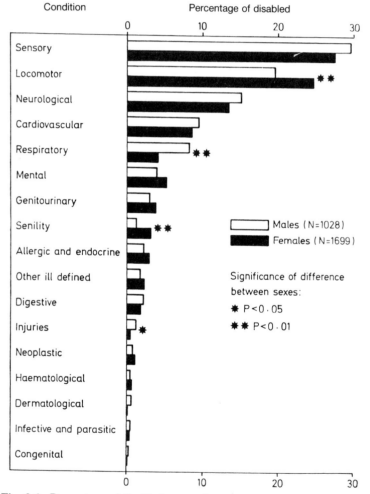

Fig. 2.1. Percentage of disabled respondents by sex and category of main disabling condition.

and women. Sensory conditions were most prevalent for both sexes (28.3 per cent). Women reported significantly more loco-motor conditions, mainly arthritic diseases, and more conditions associated with senility. Men reported significantly more respiratory conditions and more injuries. In addition to being older and female, the disabled respondents also were more likely to be widowed, separated, or divorced, not working (but of working

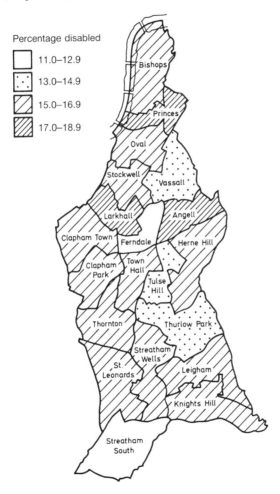

Fig. 2.2. Estimated prevalence of disabled persons in Lambeth electoral wards.

age), living in households where the head was or had been engaged in a manual occupation, and living alone. Women and men were more likely to report disability if they were older, not married, and not working (but of working age). In addition, men who were working in a manual job or living alone were more likely to report disability. For men aged 50–64, the odds of reporting being disabled and not working were much higher than for men in any other age group.

Fig. 2.2 shows that the prevalence estimates of disability across the 20 electoral wards in Lambeth ranged from 11.5 to 18.6 per cent. Two major factors accounting for this variation are the distribution of age and sex across the wards. These factors do not explain all the variation, however. Those wards with lower prevalence rates (11–13 per cent) can be characterized in two broad types: areas of more recently immigrated families with young children who are living in crowded council housing or public housing, and areas of more established families who were born in the UK and live in private households. Wards with higher prevalence rates (17–19 per cent) are areas where more people live alone or with fewer young persons, are unemployed, and/or reside in public housing that either lacks or shares use of a bath. A low response rate from the areas with higher proportions of immigrant populations may well account for the lower prevalence estimates in these areas, but no clear trend emerged. Some electoral wards are composed of households with widely varying characteristics, indicating that a smaller unit of observation may be needed to obtain a clearer picture of the association between the rates of disablement and socio–demographic, housing, environmental, or employment factors.

Disablement definitions and prevalence

The definition of disability used in the Lambeth screening study included a wider range and number of functional limitations and activity restrictions than had been used previously in many surveys. Eleven of the 25 items, however, were similar to those used in the national OPCS survey that produced prevalence estimates of 6.7 per cent for males, 8.8 per cent for females, and 7.8 per cent for all persons aged 16 and over. Prevalence estimates for the Lambeth sample based on the same 11 items were 5.9 per cent for males, 9.7 per cent for females, and 7.9 per cent for all persons. The prevalence estimates are remarkably similar, indicating that the additional limitations or restrictions in the Lambeth study were primarily responsible for the two-fold increase in prevalence.

Sensory motor items such as frequent falls and occupation-related items such as difficulty doing the job of choice or housework significantly increased reported disability. Using criteria based on ambulation, mobility, and self-care items alone would have missed a large number of potentially handicapped. By focusing simply on self-care criteria, researchers miss those who may not be severely or appreciably handicapped in self-care, but are unable to perform household activities, undertake light employment, or join social activities.

The prevalence estimates in Lambeth also were comparable to those reported in the US Health Interview Survey. This similarity arises because both sets of estimates are based on a definition of disability that emphasizes the performance of major activities appropriate for age, in particular the activities of paid work or housework.

The wording of Lambeth survey items in terms of actual 'performance' of activities rather than the 'capacity' to perform them (e.g. 'Do you have difficulty?' *versus* 'Are you able?') also influenced prevalence rates. Performance-related wording can significantly increase the reporting of difficulties on disability surveys. A comparison of the response to specific items used in both the 1968 and 1978 Lambeth health surveys allowed an examination of the effect of questionnaire wording. In 1968, the items were asked as questions about the capacity of respondents to perform activities of daily living, for example, 'Can you get in and out of bed by yourself?' or 'Can you dress or undress yourself?'. In 1978, the same questions were asked in terms of the performance or non-performance of activities because of illness, for example, 'Do you have difficulty dressing or undressing without help because of illness?'. Based on data from both surveys, the use of capacity-related wording can produce 15–20 per cent 'under-reporting' in self-reports of health status in population surveys (Anderson *et al.* 1984). Significantly higher responses to the disability items obtained in the later Lambeth survey support the importance of questionnaire wording.

Duckworth (1983) points out that assessing eligibility for financially rewarding social security benefits must be based on self-reported capacity because capacity is the concept most compatible with the provision of benefits or services. Since people tend to overestimate their ability to perform daily activities, however, observation of actual behaviour is the most valid and reliable measure of capacity. Health examination surveys of impairment have long included tests of motor skills, lung function, or vision and hearing to validate self-reports of capacity or behaviour (Jeffreys *et al.* 1969).

The type of wording to be used in a self-reported, disability survey depends upon the objective of the survey. If the objective is to identify people in a community with observable activity restrictions or functional limitations, then performance-related wording is preferable. Prevalence estimates based on the performance-related wording of disability questions will be higher than if capacity-related wording is used. On the other hand, if the objective is to estimate 'felt or expressed need', such as eligibility for disability benefits or demand for services, capacity-related wording will yield lower estimates. Reports of actual behaviours are objective statements that require less judgment on the part of the respondents. Self-reports of the performance of activities are also likely to be more reliable than self-assessed capacity.

Because persons with significant functional limitations and activity restrictions form a relatively small proportion of the community (15–20 per cent at most), a large number of households need to be surveyed in order to yield sufficient numbers of disabled people to report prevalence estimates with narrow confidence limits. Cost may be an important consideration, however. Substantial savings can be made by employing postal survey methodologies. The cost of obtaining a completed questionnaire by interview is almost double the cost of obtaining one by mail, and the cost increases with the number of stages that need to be employed to obtain an acceptable response rate of 85 per cent or higher. The one-stage, postal survey strategy for identification and prevalence estimation is a desirable alternative for many communities.

Using prevalence data for planning service provision

Prevalence estimates of disability can be used for planning health and social services in a community in two major ways. They can be used to evaluate the criteria upon which the need for health and social services is based, and they can provide information for comparing the geographical distribution of services to that of the disabled population.

The Lambeth Department of Social Services uses a measure for assessing 'handicapped' that is more general than the OPCS measure described earlier. People are classified as (1) very severely handicapped if they are housebound by virtue of a physical or mental disorder, such that they cannot get beyond their house and garden without help; or (2) severely or appreciably handicapped if they require personal assistance or social services, or are at 'risk' by virtue of their disability (Clifford 1982). The second category involves a great deal of discretion, although the notion of permanent, (i.e., irreversable) and substantial (i.e., severe), disability is used in making the determination. The Lambeth screening study's definition of handicapped, which encompasses a broader range of items, expands the definition to include limitations in major social activity. This enlarged perspective is particularly relevant to the need for home-care services such as meal preparations, shopping, doing routine chores, or handling money.

After the Lambeth study estimates were updated to the 1981 census, the local authority concluded that between 16,000 and 20,000 residents of the borough were likely to need the kind of support that it offers. About 8,700 adults are registered as physically handicapped, 79 per cent of whom are 65 years or older. The number of registered young adults represented less than a quarter of those who were estimated by the survey to need one or more of the authority's services. The number of registered elderly people, however, represented a much higher proportion of those estimated to be in need.

The factors associated with disability in Lambeth suggest that a number of groups in urban areas are more likely to report disability: persons who are older, not married, or not working (but under retirement age), especially men aged 50–64, and older men in manual occupations who live alone. Such information is helpful because it identifies client groups using criteria other than age, which is not always the most accurate measure of need. The needs of disabled people under age 16 and over age 65, for example, are believed to be so much greater than those in intermediate age groups that the latter groups receive the lowest allocation of man hours in many health and social services departments. It could be argued, however, that those persons, being of employable age, are a potentially important client group. As studies have shown, disabled persons who are unemployed, separated or divorced, or living alone need special consideration when health resources are being planned and allocated, and special efforts are required to identify their unmet needs.

Prevalence estimates among different age and sex groups by geographical distribution can reveal a mismatch between the distribution of disabled persons and the number of existing beds, clinics, or day centres. Fig. 2.3 shows the location of Lambeth's existing hospitals and day centres for the elderly and physically handicapped, compared with the distribution of disabled people over the age of 65. The number of day centres and places per elderly person in the north of the borough is clearly much greater than in the south. While residents in the south can use facilities in the north, ease of access is dependent upon the availability of transportation. Mobility limitations are common problems for physically disabled people that increase the barriers to day centre use.

This obvious mismatch between services and clients calls for more day centre services in the south of the borough. Before providing such services, however, those responsible for planning would have to consider at least four major points: (1) the objectives of day centre service for the disabled elderly, (2) the effectiveness and efficiency of current services for meeting those objectives, (3) satisfaction of the elderly with the services provided, and (4) the resources available for delivering more of the same services or alternative services.

Identifying the number of disabled people within a population and their specific disablements is an important first step for secondary and tertiary prevention (United Nations 1982). If services are to be effective, they must address actual needs. The 1978 Lambeth study showed, for example, that many residents

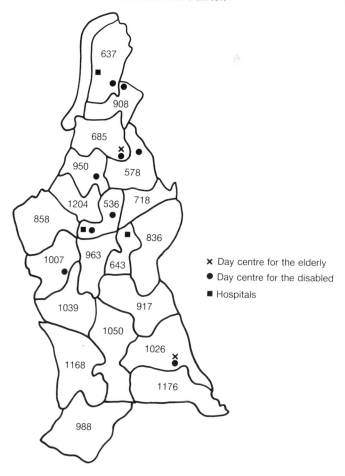

Fig. 2.3. Day centres, hospitals and number of disabled elderly persons in Lambeth by electoral wards.

have difficulties with hearing, ambulation, and locomotion. This finding suggests that the best way of helping the disabled population may be to provide more audiological services and mobility assistance. Before expanding services, however, one needs to know how many disabled people with these difficulties already receive such services, whether the services could be provided more efficiently or effectively, and whether those not receiving aids and adaptations would in fact want and be able to benefit from them (see Chapter 7).

In planning services and comparing geographical divisions, it is essential to consider factors that are known to be associated with disability. Counting the disabled and identifying high-risk groups in cross-sectional studies is only a first step in the determination of unmet needs. Planners also need information on the severity and course of disability (Chapters 3 and 4), the prospects for reducing disability through prevention (Chapters 5 and 6), the range of available and most appropriate resource strategies for rehabilitation (Chapters 7 and 8), and the willingness and ability of the community to provide care and of the disabled people to care for themselves (Chapters 9 and 10).

References

Agerholm, M. (1975). *Outset: Report London*. Outset, London.

Anderson, J., Bush, J. and Berry, C. (1984). *Performance versus capacity: a conflict in classifying function for health status measurement*. Technical Report M–022. Health Policy Projects, University of California, San Diego School of Medicine, La Jolla, California.

Bennett, A. E., Gerrard, J., and Halil, T. (1970). Chronic disease and disability in the community: a prevalence study. *British Medical Journal* **3**, 762–4.

Buckle, J. (1971). *Handicapped and impaired in Great Britain. Part II: work and housing of impaired persons in Great Britain*. HMSO, London.

Colvez, A. and Blanchet, M. (1981). Disability trends in the United States populations 1966–76: analysis of reported causes. *American Journal of Public Health* **71**, 464–71.

Clifford, B. (1982). *Physically handicapped adults in Lambeth—a review of numbers and needs*. Lambeth Social Services Directorate, London.

Duckworth, D. (1983). *The classification and measurement of disablement*. HMSO, London.

Duckworth, D. (1984). *Use of household surveys to collect statistics on disabled persons: technical report*. Statistical Office and the Centre for Social Development and Humanitarian Affairs, United Nations Secretariat, ESA STAT AC 18 3.

Harris, A. (1971). *Handicapped and impaired in Great Britain*. HMSO, London.

Harris, A. and Head, E. (1974). *Sample survey in local authority areas*.

(revised edn) Social Survey Division, Office of Population Censuses and Surveys.

Jeffreys, M., Nullard, J. B., Hyman, M., and Warren, M. D. (1969). A set of tests for measuring motor impairment in prevalence studies. *Journal of Chronic Diseases* **28**, 303–9.

Knight, R. and Warren, M. (1978). *Physically disabled people living at home: study of numbers and needs.* HMSO, London.

Locker, D., Wiggins, R., Sittampalam, Y., and Patrick, D. L. (1981). Estimating the prevalence of disability in the community: the influence of sample design and response bias. *Journal of Epidemiology and Community Health* **35**, 208–12.

National Center for Health Statistics (1986). *Health: United States, 1986.* DHSS Pub. No. (PHS) 87–1232. US Government Printing Office, Washington, DC.

National Center for Health Statistics (1981). *Data systems of the National Center for Health Statistics.* DHHS Publication No. (PHS) 82–1318, Hyattsville, Md, US, National Center for Health Statistics, US Department of Health and Human Services.

National Center for Health Statistics (1983). *Americans needing help to function at home.* DHHS Publication No. 83–1250. Hyattsville, Md.: NCHS, Public Health Service.

National Center for Health Statistics (1985). *Current estimates from the National Health Interview Survey: United States 1980.* DHHS Publication No. (PHS) 85–1578, Hyattsville, Md., US, National Center for Health Statistics, US Department of Health and Human Services.

Office of Population Census and Surveys (1983). *General Household Surveys: introductory report.* HMSO, London.

Patrick, D., Darby, S., Horton, G., Locker D., and Wiggins, R. (1981). Screening for disability in the inner city. *Journal of Epidemiology and Community Health* **35**, 65–70.

Patrick, D. L., Peach, H., and Gregg, I. (1982). Disablement and care: a comparison of patient views and general practitioner knowledge. *Journal of the Royal College of General Practitioners* **32**, 429–34.

Peach, H., Green, S., Locker, D., Darby, S., and Patrick, D. L. (1980). Evaluation of a postal screening questionnaire to identify the physically disabled. *International Rehabilitation Medicine* **2**, 189–93.

United Nations (1982). *Decade of disabled persons. 1983–92.* World Programme of action concerning disabled persons. Adopted by the United Nations General Assembly at its 37th regular session on 3 December 1982, by resolution 37/52.

US Bureau of the Census (1979). *Demographic social and economic profiles of states: Spring 1976.* Current Population Reports, Series P-20, No. 334 Government Printing Office, Washington, DC, USA.

Warren, M. D. (1974). *Canterbury survey of handicapped people.* Report

No. 6, Canterbury Health Services Research Unit, University of Kent.

Warren, M. D. (1983). *The Canterbury studies of disablement: prevalence needs services and attitudes.* Report No. 50, Canterbury, Health Services Research Unit, University of Kent.

Wing, J. K., Bebbington, P., and Robbins, L. A. (1981). *What is a case? Problems of definition in psychiatric community surveys.* Grant McIntyre, London.

Wilson, R. and Drury, T. (1984) Interpreting trends in illness and disability: health statistics and health status. *Annual Review of Public Health.* **5** 83–106.

Wood, P. H. N. and Badley, E. M. (1978). Setting disablement in perspective. *International Rehabilitation Medicine.* **1**, 32–37.

World Health Organization (WHO) (1981). *Disability prevention and rehabilitation.* Technical Report Series 668, Geneva, WHO.

3

Approaches to assessing disability

JOHN R. H. CHARLTON

Many people are better off with grave handicaps than with trifling ones. The grave handicaps release copious energies.

Walter B. Pitman, *Life Begins at Forty*

Improvements in living standards, public health measures, and modern medicine have greatly decreased the impact of infectious diseases in more developed countries, resulting in more people living longer. Unfortunately, many of these elderly people develop chronic diseases that cannot be cured, although the disabling effects of these diseases can be alleviated in some cases. As a result, doctors, community nurses, social service departments, and voluntary agencies now spend a larger proportion of their time helping patients who suffer from the disabling consequences of chronic disease. For years, charitable organizations have assisted certain disabled and disadvantaged groups such as blind and deaf people. It is only recently, however, that society has collectively taken responsibility for entire groups of people, including aging people living independently. With this added responsibility has come a greater understanding of the consequences of chronic disease and less restrictive eligibility requirements for disabled benefits. The broadening of the concept of disablement has occurred faster, however, than have discussions about who should be singled out for help and how much help they should receive. This chapter deals with methods of assessing disease consequences as a preliminary step toward deciding who is to be helped and how.

Historical development of assessing disability

The concept of disability in Britain has developed largely in conjunction with legislation for welfare provision, at a time when humanitarian concern was competing with economic constraints. The first individuals to be singled out for special help because of disease were crippled children, the blind, and the deaf. In 1893, the government established special education for blind and deaf children 'on the grounds that such children, given special training, were perfectly able to become useful citizens and workers, but left neglected would become dependent paupers' (Topliss 1979). In 1899, local education authorities were given powers to provide special schools for the 'educable mentally subnormal'. Scant attention was paid, however, to the educational needs of other physically handicapped people. The war-disabled and industrially disabled were the two groups singled out next. The consequences of their medical conditions—problems of mobility, dexterity, and employment—were assumed to be similar in type and severity for both groups so that the same principles of compensation could be applied to both. Groups that were unlikely to become useful citizens and workers, such as profoundly retarded persons or persons with quadraplegia, were largely ignored by the state and had to rely on charity.

In the National Insurance Act of 1941, differences were maintained between 'workers' and 'others', and between 'industrial disease or injury' and diseases and injuries produced by other causes. The Disabled Persons (Employment) Acts, 1944 and 1958, applied to those persons who 'on account of injury, disease, or deformity are substantially handicapped in obtaining or keeping employment, or in undertaking work on their own account, of a kind which, apart from their injury, diseases, or deformity would be suited to their age, experience, and qualifications'. Eligibility for help was expanded in 1948 by the National Assistance Act, which gave local authorities responsibility for providing accommodation and welfare services for people in their area who required it on account of age, infirmity, and other circumstances. Here the handicapped were 'those persons who are blind, deaf, or dumb, and other persons who are substantially and permanently handicapped by illness, injury, or congenital deformity, or such other disabilities as may be prescribed by the minister'. It was not clear how the 'handicapped' were to be identified or how handicap was to be measured in order to single out those who were 'substantially or permanently' affected.

There was a further widening of the eligibility criteria in the Chronically Sick and Disabled Persons Act, 1970. The Act was designed to help families cope with their appreciably or severely handicapped members for as long as possible, in an effort to keep the handicapped from having to enter institutions. The unemployable disabled were treated in the same way as the employable in this Act, and local authorities were required to provide facilities and services where previously they had been empowered only to provide these if they so wished. The act made no distinction between the needs of 'the disabled' and 'the chronically sick' since by then most disability was caused by progressive or fluctuating conditions such as cardiac disease, arthritis, or mental illness, rather than by relatively permanent conditions such as blindness. This legislation was based on the results of the national survey by the Office of Population Censuses and Surveys, which basically defined levels of handicap according to difficulties in self-care and mobility as described in Chapter 2 (Harris 1971).

This brief review of legislation concerning disablement in Britain illustrates changing views of what constitutes disability and what the 'needs' of disabled people are. Priorities for providing help were set on the basis of those thought to be most in 'need', with a gradual broadening of the eligibility criteria to more and more groups. As more legislation was enacted and more groups became entitled to benefits, increased attention was paid to the concept of disability and its assessment.

What should be assessed?

A number of authors have attempted to place the definitions and assessments of disease consequences on a firm scientific footing rather than rely on the vagaries of historical usage. This approach is especially important since there are many definitions used in different countries and within the same country, making communication and equitable provision difficult. If terms are not clearly defined, then money and services may not be directed where they are needed most and may be used for unintended purposes.

Townsend (1967) listed five aspects that need to be considered in assessing disability. The first is the physiological or psychological abnormality or loss. The second is the nature of the underlying clinical condition that alters or interrupts the normal physiological or psychological processes. These two concepts tend to merge, for although a loss may be sustained without an underlying disease, chronic disease usually has some psychological affects or limits activities of daily life such as walking, negotiating stairs, washing, and dressing. Third, limitations can occur in other aspects of ordinary life. By refering to the average person of the same age and sex, an estimate can be made of the individual's relative incapacity in, for example, household management and performance of social roles. Townsend's fourth point is that some activities are not only limited but also different. This difference may depend as much on how the limitations are perceived by the individual and his or her response to other's expectations, as on their physiological determination. Finally, the socially-defined position or status of the individual needs to be considered. The chronically sick person may occupy a status that attracts a mixture of deference, condescension, consideration, or indifference. Regardless of a disabled individual's specific behaviour or condition, he or she attracts attention from the rest of the population by virtue of the position that chronically sick people occupy in society. These five aspects are of variable importance depending on the purpose of disablement assessment.

Purposes of disablement assessment

There are a number of possible approaches to measuring and assessing disability. The most appropriate method to choose will depend upon the following purposes of the assessment:

1. *Planning.* Those planning the provision of services, aids, and housing for people with disabilities may need only counts or estimates of disabled people according to an appropriate definition, with types of disability classified and possibly ranked on a crude index of severity.

2. *Monitoring patient care.* Those involved with the rehabilitation of individuals need to monitor closely the progress of each patient in a number of areas of life, such as mobility, social interaction, and emotional behaviour, in order to gain a better understanding of how further intervention is most likely to benefit the patient.

3. *Evaluating interventions.* Researchers and clinicians may wish to use randomized controlled trials to compare the effectiveness of different programmes of care, for example, different regimes of physiotherapy or counselling. The routine monitoring of patients and the evaluation of intervention strategies both require sophisticated instruments capable of quantifying change in the various aspects of disablement. Measures that are specific to the intervention are desirable as outcome measures, although more global measures also are useful to give an indication of the intervention's overall effect.

4. *Epidemiology.* Epidemiological studies of the causes and course of disablement also require reliable and valid measures sensitive to changes in the status of impairment, disability, and handicap.

5. *Assessing eligibility for benefits.* The process whereby individuals are assessed to determine their eligibility for State benefits can be regarded as measurement, at least in the sense of being more or less 'eligible'. In practice, eligibility does not necessarily relate closely to the level of functioning in the individual. The Disability Alliance (1975) has suggested that 'functional' criteria based on specific disabilities could provide a rational and widely applicable method for assessing disability. Sainsbury (1974) has developed a method based on such functional criteria, in this case the incapacity to perform certain activities associated with daily living. Townsend (1979) has argued that the use of a functional measure of disability might lead to a distribution of resources that is fairer than the present one.

Duckworth (1983) discusses in detail the assessment of disablement within social security practice. He favours graded assessments, which relate amount of benefit to degree of disability whenever it is feasible. This practice has the advantage of reducing the chance of improperly classifying closely adjacent categories, such as minimally and moderately disabled. Some graded assessment does occur when compensation is made for industrial injuries and war-disablement pensions. Once eligibility has been established in such pensions, the degree of disablement is assessed in percentage terms. Rudimentary objective instruments exist for aiding assessment and for reducing variability between assessors (Department of Health and Social Security 1970, 1976). Claimants also might be better served if the social and psychosocial effects of impairment were part of the assessment. This issue raises the question of who should be the assessor. If impairments are the targets of measurement, then a medical practitioner would be the most appropriate arbiter. If disability or even handicap are to be the basis for compensation, however, then other professionals are likely to be involved along with disabled persons.

Criteria for choosing a disability measure

In discussing the choice of health status indicators, of which impairment, disability, and handicap are components, Jette (1980) has suggested that four points need to be considered. These are: (1) the intended use of the measure, for example, to compare two treatments, to see if provision of services matches 'needs', or to monitor individual patients over time; (2) the conceptual focus, for example, whether impairment, disability, or handicap, or all three, are to be measured; (3) the quality of the measures, such as their validity, reliability, sensitivity to changes; and (4) the operational approach, for example, whether information is to be gathered by questionnaire, by professional assessors, or from routine sources, or abstracted from records. Jette's paper provides a useful comparison of about a dozen indicators relevant to chronic disease evaluation reseach. In the area of health status assessment, the term 'indicator' is used to describe a single measure of population morbidity or mortality, and 'index' refers to several indicators combined. The reliability and validity of any indicator or index and the practicability of using them are important aspects when considering whether to use particular instruments, even though few instruments have been evaluated extensively.

Broadly speaking, the validity of an instrument is the extent to which the instrument measures what it purports to measure. Reliability is concerned with the accuracy or repeatability of the instrument, for example, whether different observers will obtain the same result. Ware *et al.* (1981) think that of all the qualities of an instrument, face validity (whether the instrument appears to measure what it is meant to, when judged by experts) is the most important factor when choosing a measure. In choosing an index, it is important to be convinced that the instrument provides information that closely matches the user's objectives. The user may wish to measure a broad range of impairments, disabilities, and handicaps, or just concentrate on a few restricted aspects; it may be pointless or even misleading to measure more than is required.

A further issue in choosing measures of disablement for evaluating interventions is whether global or more intervention-specific indices should be used. Global indices combine different aspects of disability, such as walking, self-care, and mobility, into a single measure or score, while specific indicators or profiles of indicators keep those aspects separate. While it may not be desirable to lose potentially valuable information by combining different observations when monitoring the progress of an individual patient, using a smaller set of global indexes in surveys may have the following advantages:

1. Disability can be summarized using a smaller number of scores, thus aiding analysis and presentation.
2. The repeatability of the scores is often increased.
3. The usefulness of scores in identifying disabled people is increased when the items are combined. Individual score distributions are usually highly skewed, and scores that apply to fewer than one per cent of the study population, for instance, would be of minimal use in testing hypotheses dealing with the effect of changes in medical care on health status, unless very large numbers of people are included in a study.
4. A more global instrument often has greater precision when used to test certain hypotheses, such as the theory that greater disability leads to greater use of medical or social services.
5. The use of a smaller set of measures helps simplify the instrument.

If the researcher uses a global instrument, which combines information from several areas of life into one score, the relative importance of the different aspects will need to be weighted. For example, in evaluating an intervention where symptoms may improve but side-effects will result, the investigator will have to decide on the relative importance of each aspect. Harris (1971) and others who have used activities of daily living (ADL) measures have themselves assigned scores to items, while others such as Patrick *et al.* (1973), Bergner *et al.* (1981), Hunt and

McEwan (1980) and Rosser and Kind (1978) have employed panels of judges to assess the relative disadvantages of different health status items and create the appropriate scores.

The construction of global measures can be criticized for obscuring impairment changes in the individual, thus making the measures of doubtful reliability and validity. Krischer (1979) has shown mathematically that measures derived by summing severity scores for combinations of health status items are valid only if the relative severity of any two states is not altered by the presence or absence of a third. Of the global scales we will review, only the scale developed by Rosser and Kind (1978) is not based on this assumption, but their instrument is comparatively simple, combining an eight-level 'disability' (dependency) scale with a four-level 'distress' scale. Here the relative severity of different disability states was found to depend on the level of distress. Although the information lost in combining measures may be important when assessing individuals, it is unlikely to be important for survey purposes as will be demonstrated in Chapter 4. From a practical point of view, any instrument which provides useful information and is simple to apply and score is more likely to be used. Again, the relative merits of any type of instrument will depend specifically upon the intended application.

In this volume, the primary focus is on assessing disability for planning health and social policy. A thorough understanding of the problems of disablement requires the quantification of each of the aspects outlined by Townsend (1967): the disease itself, its manifestation, the way it restricts the individual's activities, and the resulting disadvantages and social stigma. For particular planning purposes a restricted range of disease consequences may be measured because there may be little point in measuring consequences outside the control of the planning authority. The data will need to be gathered by questionnaire, which could be self-completed or interviewer-administered, since it is unlikely that appropriate routine data will exist and professional assessment may be too expensive. Validity will have to be established to prevent biased estimates, and the reliability will have to be adequate enough for the study's purposes. Different measures of disablement are reviewed briefly in the following section.

The International Classification of Impairment, Disability, and Handicap (ICIDH)

As reviewed in Chapter 1, the ICIDH assesses losses, chronic disease, functional limitations (impairments), behavioural changes (disabilities), and the disadvantages experienced by people in survival roles as a result of impairment (handicaps). These aspects of disease consequences have different implications for intervention services. Medical and paramedical services generally help to prevent impairments from causing disability, while social services help to prevent the handicapping consequences of disabilities. The international classification system does not deal explicitly, however, with the social stigma associated with chronic conditions.

In theory, handicap is the most crucial aspect to assess in order to determine need for resources. If the disabled individual is not disadvantaged, there is little justification for further intervention. Once handicap has been established, however, it is essential to know more about the precursors of that handicap, in other words, to assess the nature and degree of impairment and disability. Seven parallel dimensions of handicap are defined in the ICIDH: orientation, physical independence, mobility, occupation, social integration, economic self-sufficiency, and other. A profile for an individual can be derived when all three codes, impairments (I), disability (D), and handicap (H), which are meant to be exhaustive, are used in conjunction with the International Classification of Disease (ICD).

While the I and D classifications describe distinct aspects, the survival roles comprising the handicap classification describe overlapping areas of life, for example, occupation and economic self-sufficiency. It has been suggested that the I-code would probably be used as an indicator of unmet needs or as a classification of health-related problems that an individual is likely to encounter. The D-code would present a profile of the individual's functional abilities, as determined from the disabilities present. By describing the physical and social environment of an individual, it is possible to match an individual's capacities with his or her environment, for example, to assist in job placement and vocational rehabilitation.

The D-code has two optional, additional digits that can be used to quantify disability. The first allows for a global assessment of the severity of disability, and the second for an assessment of prognosis. Seven arbitrary grades of severity are specified in increasing order of severity: not disabled (0), difficulty in performance (1), aided performance (2), assisted performance (3), dependent performance (4), augmented inability (5), and complete inability (6). These grades correspond to seven intervention goals: enhancement of performance (relating to grade 1), supplementation by use of aids or human help (grades 2–4), and substitution of activity by another person (grades 5–6). Seven grades of prognosis also are suggested, ranging from not disabled (0) to deteriorating disability (6). Coding difficulties arise if an individual has several disabilities of varying severity, some of which interact.

The H-code indicates the extent to which an individual's potential is realized, and each of the survival roles is graded according to degree of disadvantage. Handicap is related to the culture in which the individual lives. Three major problems emerge in using the classification of handicap. First, disadvantage may be perceived in three ways: subjectively by the individual; by others who are significant to the individual; and by the community as a whole. A choice has to be made as to which of these perceptions should be used. Second, there is ambiguity over how to regard third-party handicaps, such as a handicapped individual who is not impaired but who suffers disadvantage because of the demands made upon him or her by chronic illness or disability in the family. Third, it is not possible for any such scheme for international use to correspond closely with any particular country's eligibility criteria for various benefits.

Duckworth (1983) has discussed the possibility of using the ICIDH for assessing disabilities in household surveys. As yet no national household interview surveys have been conducted that use the ICIDH classification system or definitions precisely. Data collection by household survey place severe limitations on the quantity of data that can be collected, and questionnaire instruments need to be extremely simple and straightforward, which precludes the use of the full ICIDH classification. Duckworth (1984) suggests that the ICIDH conceptual scheme could be used as a basis for surveys administered by trained interviewers. In a highly simplified form it would be useful for establishing the prevalence of different types of disabilities among individuals and, possibly, for describing severity and prognosis. The classification was not designed for this purpose, however, and valid and reliable instruments based on it would need to be developed. Conceptual and methodological problems have been encountered in attempts to use the ICIDH in health assessment surveys (Colvez and Robine, 1986; de Kleijn-de Vrankrijker, 1986). The ICIDH lacks exact description and criteria for coding as well as practical tools for survey use.

Activities of daily living measures

There are many instruments for assessing loss of independence in the activities of daily living (ADL), which are used by occupational therapists and others in rehabilitation medicine to monitor the progress of treatment or to assess the outcome. Some ADL scales have been used in surveys (Katz *et al.* 1983). These scales define activities an individual should be able to perform unaided. The questionnaire used by Harris (1971) consisted of 9 items of daily living, with emphasis on personal care. A further group of measures, called instrumental activities of daily living (IADL), assess more complex activities such as ability to cook, shop, or use public transportation. While provider ratings tend to agree with patient self-reported ratings on the simple ADL items, this is not necessarily the case for the more complex self-care activities.

Many of the ADL instruments have not been thoroughly tested for reliability and validity. These instruments have been reviewed in the literature, by Bruett and Overs (1969) for example, who described twelve such indices. There are three basic types. The first type of ADL measure lists the disabilities and is designed to measure the effectiveness of overall treatment, preferably by means of a single score. For those instruments it is essential to devise some kind of scoring system so that information describing different activity restrictions can be combined. Andrews (1976) has criticized these attempts, because no standardized approach has been used and because a great deal of potentially valuable information may be lost in forming a single score. The same score for 2 patients or even the same patient on two occasions may sometimes obscure large differences in the pattern of disabilities experienced. Kelman and Willner (1962) have examined the repeatability of such measures, and they conclude that the same population measured by different, but equally qualified examiners, under different test conditions, yielded different results. This irregularity could be influenced by changes in environment, observer differences, lack of standardization of methods, and the natural variability of the patients being measured.

The second type of ADL measure yields profiles that are not averaged or totalled to describe the activities patients can perform. Smith *et al.* (1977) have designed an instrument that is suitable for making reliable home assessments while the patient is still undergoing hospital treatment. They suggest that each patient be scored on a grid where category '1' is completely independent, '2' is independent using prescribed aids, '3' requires supervision for safety but no physical help, and so on with category '7' being completely dependent. There are similarities between Smith's categories and the seven suggested in the ICIDH, which could be used as an alternative grading.

While most British ADL indices have not been validated carefully, the ADL measures developed by Katz and Akpom (1976), in the USA, have been extensively tested for reliability and validity. They identified a set of activities (feeding, continence, transferring from bed, toileting, dressing, bathing), which are more or less cumulatively related to one another in severity. Guttman scaling (Guttman 1950) was employed to derive scores based on the number of areas of dependency in ADL. These scores were developed using samples covering a wide range of chronically sick and disabled people, including children and mentally impaired adults. Inter-user reliability is high, with trained users differing only 5 per cent of the time.

The third type of ADL index consists of a long, usually non-additive list of items, with as many items as are necessary to record all activities. This type of index is discussed by Oppenheim (1966) who suggests that it is at its best when constructed to test specific hypotheses rather than to serve as an exploratory tool. Many such instruments have not been adequately piloted and are of doubtful validity. Thus they should be considered critically before being used.

Great Britain's OPCS National Survey

The 9-item questionnaire used in the 1969 national survey

conducted by the Office of Population Censuses and Surveys (OPCS/NS) was based almost exclusively on self-care activities and incorporated a set of weights arbitrarily chosen to reflect severity (Harris 1971). The OPCS/NS measure was divided into major items (feeding, getting to or using the toilet, doing up buttons and zips) and minor items (putting on shoes and socks, other dressing, bathing and all over wash, washing face and hands, getting in and out of bed, and shaving for men or combing/brushing hair for women). 'Generally having difficulty doing' a major item resulted in a score of four, and a minor item netted a score of two. Inability to do an item scored six for a major item and three for a minor item. Scores were calculated and graded subjectively into five grades: no disability (0), minor (2–5), appreciable (6–11), severe (12–17), and very severe (19–36).

This study has been criticized for the narrowness of its definition of disability, and for the lack of a statistical or explicit value-weighting scheme for the items. Bebbington (1977), however, has shown, with data from a survey in Kingston, that four different methods of scaling the severity of the OPCS/NS survey items produce essentially the same results for groups of individuals. He concludes that the choice of scoring weights is often irrelevant, provided the scale consists of a number of similar items, each with a small number of clearly ordered categories. The result is a unidimensional scale. Any scale that is suitable for Guttman scaling (i.e., has a high coefficient of reproducibility) will have those properties, and it is probably unnecessary to consider more sophisticated weighting systems. Duckworth (1983), based on his experiences with an instrument similar to the OPCS/NS measure, also found that the overall distribution of disability scores was altered little by the actual values chosen for the severity weights in an additive scale. Measures formed from larger sets of items often do not form a unidimensional scale, particularly if a wider set of disease consequences than self-care or mobility is to be measured. For those more comprehensive measures, different approaches to scoring systems or severity weighting produce different results (Bush 1984).

Health status indices

A large number of health status indices have been developed and tested for reliability and validity, based on different types of measurement (McDowell and Newell, 1987). To date, an instrument designed specifically to measure all five of Townsend's concepts does not exist, but available health status instruments that are based primarily on capacity for or performance of daily activities can be adapted for use as indices of disability. Among the health status instruments that might be considered for measuring disablement are the Nottingham Health Profile (Hunt and McEwan 1980), the US National Health Interview Survey measure (National Center for Health Statistics 1975), the Quality of Well-Being Scale (Patrick *et al.* 1973), the Sickness Impact Profile (Bergner *et al.* 1981), those developed for the Rand Health Insurance Experiment in the US (Brook *et al.* 1983); and a scale developed by Rosser and Kind (1978).

The Nottingham Health Profile was designed as a simple, standardized, self-administered measure of perceived physical, social, and mental health problems. It was intended to serve as an indicator of population health status and to provide some assessment of a person's need for care. However it was not based purely on medical criteria, thus enabling the subsequent evaluation of the care provided for such persons. It comprises two parts. Part one consists of 38 statements grouped into six areas: pain, physical mobility, sleep, energy, social isolation, and emotional reactions. These statements were formulated on the basis of interviews with 768 patients who had a variety of acute and chronic ailments. Each item has a severity weight, which was determined by the method of paired comparisons. The weights were estimated subjectively by a sample of people drawn from patient and non-patient groups. When the instrument is administered, the respondent endorses the items that apply to him or her, and the weights corresponding to those items are added to produce scores for each of the six areas of life. Part two was designed to give a general estimate of those areas of social functions perceived to be affected by the health problems of the individual. It comprises a single yes/no statement on each of the following areas: paid employment, jobs around the home, social life, sex life, family relationships, hobbies/interests, and holidays. The profile has been tested for validity where it has been found to compare favourably with other health status indicators. The individual items making up the profile, however, reflect both impairment and disability. Investigators may wish to separate those aspects, since the implications for intervention at each level of disablement differ.

The US National Health Interview Survey, conducted annually on a national sample, assesses the presence of illness and injury and describes acute and chronic conditions and related disability in terms of restricted activity, bed disability, and work and school-loss days caused by the condition. It also assesses the degree of duration of activity limitations (National Center for Health Statistics 1975). Those broad measures provide useful information on disability and its trends over time (Colvez and Blanchet 1981).

The Quality of Well-Being Scale (QWB) (Patrick *et al.* 1973; Kaplan and Bush 1980) was developed to measure attributes of function and symptom/problem complexes. Each item is an objectively reportable fact that occurred on a given day, including institutionalization, self-care, social activities, driving/public transportation, walking, and bed disability. The QWB combines health-related quality of life with mortality, includes a method of estimating prognosis, and has severity weights that have been obtained from explicit value-scaling studies. The final comprehensive outcome expression is Well-Life Expectancy, which integrates the expected duration (quantity) with the expected quality of life computed from the observed transition between levels of wellness. The QWB has been tested extensively for validity and reliability, and it has been applied in a number of chronic disease evaluations, including a clinical trial of chronic obstructive pulmonary disease (Kaplan *et al.* 1984), as well as in other health evaluations. The QWB lacks a significant component scale in mental health and yields only an overall score rather than a series of separate scales with an overall score. Because of the complexity of the measurement model and the global index score provided by the QWB, the measure may be more suitable for assessing population health status than for use in chronic disease and disability studies on specific populations.

In addition to condition-specific measures of physiological health and measures of health habits, the Rand Health Insurance Experiment developed survey measures of five general health status concepts: physical and role functioning, mental health, social well-being, and general health perception (Brook *et al.* 1983). This comprehensive battery of health status measures was derived mainly from previous work in the field, although the Rand investigators have investigated their scales extensively using factor analysis, and validity, reliability, and stability studies. Of particular interest is the General Health Rating Index comprising 22 statements of opinions about personal health (Davies and Ware 1981). This index discriminates between those with and without a chronic disease such as arthritis or hypertension. It is sensitive to individual differences in disease severity and to changes in both physical and mental functioning. Such a general scale of health perceptions may be a useful supplement to the function status and ADL measures used in many disability studies.

Sickness Impact Profile

Another health status instrument, which focuses on the performance of usual activities but also covers some symptoms, is the Sickness Impact Profile (SIP) (Bergner *et al.* 1981). The SIP was developed in Seattle with funding from the United States Government to provide a measure that is broadly applicable across types and severity of illness and across demographic and cultural sub-groups, yet sensitive enough to detect changes or differences in health status that may occur over time or between groups. SIP items were obtained from over 1,200 statements describing the behavioural impacts of sickness; for example: 'I am walking shorter distances'; or 'I sit around half asleep'. These statements were collected from patients in out-patient and other clinics, predominately from a prepaid group practice. The results were subjected to standard grouping and sorting techniques, yielding 312 unique items. Further field trials were conducted to reduce the number of items. In its final form the SIP comprises 136 yes/no statements, almost all of which refer to restrictions in activity, and which cover a broader spectrum of daily activities than do most other available instruments. The items are grouped into 12 sets or categories that assess the impact of sickness on different areas of daily life by means of 12 scores, each of which is the weighted sum of the statements that an individual considers applicable to him or herself. The SIP can be self-completed, interviewer-administered, or based on the proxy reports of others. The weights for the items were obtained using the psychometric technique of category-scaling (Carter *et al.* 1976) which involves a sample of people judging the severity of individual items and assigning to each a severity category. Physician, nurses, and health administration students, who judged the SIP items to determine the severity weights, agreed highly on the relative severity of dysfunction represented by each item.

The SIP scores have been assessed for validity by comparing them with: self-reports of dysfunction and sickness; clinician reports of patient dysfunction and severity of illness; and with other measures of dysfunction or sickness, such as T4 for hyperthyroidism and the Harris Analysis of Hip Function for hip replacement patients. Good convergent and discriminant validity has been reported (Bergner 1984). The 24-hour, test–retest reliability is approximately 0.90 for the entire instrument, and the internal consistency reliability is approximately 0.80. The SIP has been used in a wide variety of applications, primarily in clinical trials and in other biomedical research.

Functional Limitations Profile

The SIP was chosen for adaptation in the Lambeth studies of disablement because of its comprehensive descriptions, its logical fit with disablement concepts, and its demonstrated reliability, validity, and sensitivity. While the 136 items make the instrument lengthy to administer, the SIP met the need for comprehensive and tested measures to compare and evaluate individuals with varying types and degrees of dysfunction, using a household interview survey. Because the categories of sickness behaviour for the US SIP items were obtained and applied in a general population in the US, it was possible to investigate the content and relevance of each item for conformity to British English usage (Patrick 1981). Whenever necessary, items were re-worded to make them more meaningful to the British population. The modified SIP, called the Functional Limitations Profile (FLP), was tested in a pilot study using patients in a general practice in England (Kingston-upon-Thames) (Patrick *et al.* 1982).

The 136 SIP statements were assigned scale values that reflect the severity of dysfunction as judged by a group of consumers and health professionals in Seattle, Washington. To investigate possible cultural differences between British and American populations, a partial replication scaling study was conducted in Lambeth to compare SIP and FLP scale values using a sample of individuals from Lambeth as judges. A two-step, equal-interval scaling procedure was used. In the first session, judges rated items within each FLP category by indicating how 'dysfunctional' they considered each item to be for the particular category of behaviour. The second step involved comparing the least and most dysfunctional items across the different categories to provide anchor weights for the scaling of all items. The Lambeth values were highly predictive of the Seattle values, indicating that the judges gave strikingly similar ratings to the items (Patrick *et al.* 1985).

On the FLP, respondents are asked whether each statement describes them 'today' and if so, whether the condition described is due to their health. If the answer to both questions is 'yes', then the severity weight associated with the item contributes to the respondent's disability scores. A score is calculated for each category by adding the scale values of all the items checked within that category by the respondent and by dividing by the maximum possible disability score for that category (see Appendix 2). This figure is then multiplied by 100 to obtain the category score. Similarly, the overall FLP score is calculated by adding the scale values for each item checked across all categories and by dividing by the maximum possible disability score for the FLP. Dysfunction also can be described in terms of five global scores rather than twelve (Charlton *et al.* 1983). Those scores represent physical disability, psychosocial disability, eating disability, communication disability, and work disability.

Jette (1980) has criticized the SIP as a generic index of health because it provides poor coverage of feeling states and does not cover physical signs. He also believes the SIP lacks measurement sensitivity because it neglects the range of performance between the ability or inability to perform activities, and because it provides limited attention to the more subjective components of performance such as pain or trouble. The SIP, however, is one of the most comprehensive health status measures with great relevance for both the clinician and the patient. It is particularly appropriate for examining the impact of impairment on the chronically ill, since it is possible to link specific medical performance to specific functional limitations and activity restrictions (see Chapter 5).

Comparison of FLP with local authority grading of disability
During the second round of interviews in the Lambeth Health

Survey, investigators included questions that enabled them to calculate the grades of disability which the Department of Health and Social Security had recommended that local authorities use in estimating the need for services for the disabled in their respective areas (Harris 1971). Comparison of the OPCS/NS measure with the FLP has yielded information on the functioning of the 1969 OPCS/NS instrument, as well as provided a means of comparing that established self-care measure with the FLP (Somerville *et al.* 1983). The OPCS/NS National Survey measure is based almost exclusively on self-care, whereas the FLP assesses the severity of restriction in a much wider range of activities.

Table 3.1 shows the correspondence between classifications of respondents on the OPCS/NS and FLP measures. Twenty eight per cent of the sample was classified as severely disabled when assessed on the FLP, compared with only 5 per cent when assessed on the OPCS/NS measure. Respondents who had low OPCS/NS scores, but high FLP scores, were compared on a number of criteria, including their FLP category scores and their use of services with those who had high OPCS/NS scores. The FLP

Table 3.1. *Office of Population, Censuses, and Surveys National Survey (OPCS/NS)*

Number of disabled people in FLP severity grades of disability

OPCS/NS grade	FLP grade			Percentage in all FLP grades	Percentage in each OPCS/NS grade
	'Low'	Moderate to appreciable	'High' severe/very severe		
'Low' OPCS/NS	336	177	126	639	(86)
Appreciable OPCS/NS	5	15	49	69	(9)
'High' Severe/very severe OPCS/NS	0	6	34	40	(5)
All OPCS/NS grades	341	198	209	748	(100)
Percentage in each FLP grade	(46)	(26)	(28)	(100)	

profiles of the 'Low OPCS/NS/High FLP' group and the 'High OPCS/NS' group were not significantly different at conventional levels, except for higher scores in the body care and movement categories in the 'High OPCS/NS' group. Thus differences between the two groups are not due solely to the psychological and social disabilities included in the FLP. On the average, the two groups have similar disabilities for ambulation, mobility, and household management, all of which are conventionally accepted aspects of disability.

The two groups were broadly similar in terms of medical conditions, and 85 per cent of the 'Low OPCS/NS/High FLP' group reported having had appreciable disability 12 months previously (FLP over 12), indicating that they were likely to have long-term rather than acute illness. Thus the OPCS/NS measure fails to identify many disabled people who may need services. This failure is largely because it does not include limitations in household management. However, local authorities vary in how they determine eligibility for services, and in Lambeth the 'Low OPCS/NS/High FLP' group included a substantial number of users of health and social services and people registered as disabled.

While the OPCS/NS measure is deficient in some aspects, the FLP, is too complex and lengthy to be used for routine local authority surveys. The FLP also measures some aspects of life that may be irrelevant to local authority services. Thus, we see it is possible for a broad, yet largely unusable instrument such as the FLP to contribute to understanding the problems of disabled people, while investigators continue to rely on an assessment measure with certain deficiences.

Clearly, we need global measures of disability that are reliable and valid, and a large number of instruments have been developed to meet this need. The FLP was developed for the Lambeth studies of disablement based on an existing instrument created in the US, which is a comprehensive and sensitive indicator of sickness-related dysfunction. The FLP has been tested in a pilot study in general practice, investigated for its measurement properties including the cross-cultural stability of its severity scoring system, and compared with an existing system of grading disability used by local authorities in the UK. Chapter 4 describes how such a disability measure can be used in a longitudinal investigation of disabled people living in the community.

References

Andrews, K. (1976). *Criteria review of the measurement of disability in the stroke patient*. Stroke Research Unit, Department of Geriatric Medicine, University of Manchester.

Bebbington, A. C. (1977). Scaling indices of disablement. *British Journal of Preventive and Social Medicine* **31**, 122–26.

Bergner, M. (1984). The Sickness Impact Profile (SIP). In *Assessment of quality of life in clinical trials of cardiovascular therapies*. (eds N. Wenger, M. E. Mattson, C. Furbert, *et al.*). LeJacq, New York.

Bergner, M., Bobbitt, R. A., Carter, W. B., and Gibson, B. S. (1981). The Sickness Impact Profile: development and final revision of a health status measure. *Medical Care* **19**, 789–805.

Brook, R., Ware, J., Rodgers, W., Keller, E., Davies, A., Donald, C., Goldberg, G., Lohr, K., Mastbay, P., and Newhouse, J. (1983). Does free care improve adults' health? Results from a randomised controlled trial. *New England Journal of Medicine* **309**, 1426.

Bruett, T. L. and Overs, R. P. (1969). A critical review of 12 ADL scales. *Physical Therapy* **49**, 857–62.

Bush, J. (1984). Relative preference versus relative frequencies in health-related quality of life evaluation. In *Assessment of quality of life in clinical trials of cardiovascular therapies*. (eds N. Wenger, M. E. Mattson, C. Furberg, *et al.*). LeJacq, New York.

Carter, W., Bobbitt, R., Bergner, M., *et al.* (1976). Validation of an interval scaling. The Sickness Impact Profile. *Health Services Research* **11**, 516–28.

Charlton, J. R. H., Patrick, D. L., and Peach. (1983). Use of multivariate measures of disability in health surveys. *Journal of Epidemiology and Community Health* **37**, 296–304.

Colvez, A. and Blanchet, M. (1981). Disability trends in the United States population 1966–76: Analysis of reported causes. *American Journal of Public Health* **71**, 464–71.

Colvez, A. and Robine, J. M. (1986). Problems encountered in using the concepts of impairment, disability, and handicap in a health assessment survey of the elderly in Upper Normandy. *International Rehabilitation Medicine* **8**, 18–22.

Davies, A. and Ware, J. (1981). *Measuring health perceptions in the health insurance experiment*. R–2711–HH3. The Rand Corporation Santa Monica, California.

de Kleijn-de Vrankrijker, M. W. (1986). Application of the ICIDH in interview surveys. *International Rehabilitation Medicine* **8**, 23–25.

Department of Health and Social Security (1970). *Handbook for war pensions medical boards*. DHSS, London.

Department of Health and Social Security (1976). *Handbook for industrial injuries medical records*. HMSO, London.

Disability Alliance (1975). *Poverty and disability*. Disability Alliance, London.

Duckworth, D. (1983). *The classification and measurement of disablement*. Research report No. 10. HMSO, London.

Duckworth, D. (1984). *Use of household surveys to collect statistics of disabled persons*. Technical report ESA/STAT/AC 18/3, Statistical Office of the United Nations Secretariat, New York.

Guttman, L. (1950). The basis for scalogram analysis. In *Measurement and prediction*. (ed S. A. Stouffer). Princetown University Press, Princetown.

Harris, A. I. (1971). *Handicapped and impaired in Great Britain. Part 1*. HMSO, London.

Hunt, S. M. and McEwan N. (1980). The development of a subjective health indicator. *Sociology of Health and Illness* **2**, 231–46.

Jette, A. M. (1980). Health status indicators: their utility in chronic disease evaluation research. *Journal of Chronic Diseases* **33**, 567–79.

Kaplan, R., Atkins, C., and Simms, R. (1984). Validity of a quality of well-being scale as an outcome measure in chronic obstructive pulmonary disease. *Journal of Chronic Diseases* **37**, 85–95.

Kaplan, R. and Bush, J. (1980). Health-related quality of life measurement for evaluation research and policy analysis. *Health Psychology* **1**, 61–80.

Katz, S. and Akpom, C. A. (1976). A measure of primary sociobiological functions. *International Journal of Health Services* **6**, 492–508.

Katz, S., Branch, L., Bronson, M., Papsidero, J., Beck, J., and Greer, D. (1983). Active life expectancy. *New England Journal of Medicine*. **309**, 1218–24.

Kelman, H. R. and Willner, A. (1962). Problems in measurement and evaluation of rehabilitation. *Archives of Physical Medicine and Rehabilitation* **43**, 177–81.

Krischer, J. P. (1979). Indexes of severity: conceptual development. *Health Services Research* **14**, 56–67.

McDowell, I. and Newell, C. (1987). *Measuring health: a guide to rating scales and questionnaires*. Oxford University Press.

National Center for Health Statistics (1975). *Health interview survey procedure 1957–74*. DHEW Publication No. (HRA) 75–1311. Department of Health, Education and Welfare, Rockville, MD, USA.

Oppenheim, A. N. (1966). *Questionnaire design and attitude measurement*. Heinemann, London.

Patrick, D. L., Bush, J. W., and Chen, M. M. (1973). Measuring levels of well-being for a health status index. *Health Services Research* **8**, 228–45.

Patrick, D. (1981). *Standardisation of comparative health status measures: using scales developed in America in an English speaking country.* Health Survey Research Methods Third Biennial Conference. Department of Health and Human Services, Hyattsville, USA.

Patrick, D. L., Peach, H., and Gregg, I. (1982). Disablement and care: a comparison of patient views and general practitioner knowledge. *Journal Royal College of General Practitioners* **32**, 429–34.

Patrick, D., Sittampalam, Y., Somerville, S. Carter, W., and Bergner, M. (1985). A cross-cultural comparison of health status values. *American Journal of Public Health* **71**(12): 1402–1407.

Rosser, R. and Kind, P. (1978). A scale of valuations of states of illness: is there a social consequent? *International Journal of Epidemiology* **7**, 347–58.

Sainsbury, S. (1974). *Measuring disability.* Occasional papers in social administration No. 54. Bell, London.

Smith, M. E., Garraway, W. M., Athtar, A. J., and Andrews, D. J. A. (1977). Measuring the outcome of stroke rehabilitation. *British Journal of Occupational Therapy* **40**(3) 51–3.

Somerville, S., Patrick, D. L., and Silver, R. (1983). Services for disabled people; what criteria should we use to assess disability? *Community Medicine* **5**, 302–10.

Topliss, E. (1979) *Provision for the disabled.* (2nd edn) Martin Robertson.

Townsend, P. (1967). *The disabled in society.* Greater London Association for the Disabled, London.

Townsend, P. (1979). *Poverty in the United Kingdom.* Penguin, Harmondsworth.

Ware, J., Brook, R. H., Davis, A. R., and Lohr, K. N. (1981). Choosing measures of health status for individuals in general populations. *American Journal of Public Health* **71**, 620–25.

4

Measuring disability in a longitudinal survey

JOHN R. H. CHARLTON

To many people science is a matter of measurements carried out with meticulous accuracy. Such measurements play a great role in developing a discovery but they are rarely its cause.

George P. Thompson, *The Inspiration of Science*

The screening study described in Chapter 2 was followed by a longitudinal disability interview survey, called the Lambeth Health Survey. This survey was conducted to provide information on the course of impairment and disability in persons living at home, and on the social situations and characteristics of disabled people that are associated with their physical, social, and psychological functioning. Included in each interview were questions describing health status and disability, socio-demographic characteristics, work, medical conditions and symptoms, social network and social support, use of health and social services, and income. Random samples of disabled and non-disabled respondents were drawn from the individuals previously screened, in such a way as to ensure that there were approximately equal numbers of men and women in the age groups 16–64 and 65–77, and that the non-disabled control group would have a similar age and sex distribution to the disabled group. For a complete description of the field methods and procedures used in the Lambeth Health Survey, see the methodological report by Ritchie and Patrick (forthcoming).

The samples

Three approximately equally spaced interviews, representing

Phases I, II, and III, were undertaken over a 2-year period. The samples are shown in Fig. 4.1. Successful interviews took place with 81 per cent of the disabled sample and 70 per cent of the control sample selected at the first phase.

The distribution of respondents at the first interview by age and sex for each of the two samples is shown in Table 4.1. The proportions of males to females was nearly matched for respon-

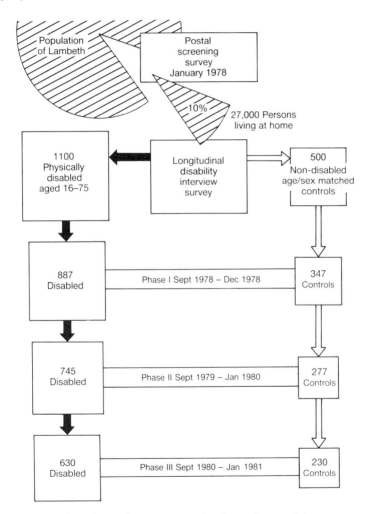

Fig. 4.1. Samples and responses to the three phases of the survey.

dents in all age groups. Within the age strata 25–44 and 45–64, the disabled sample contained higher proportions of older respondents than did the control sample. Only 5 per cent of the disabled sample were aged 16–24, compared with 15 per cent of the control sample. The marital status of disabled and non-disabled respondents was similar, the only significant difference occurring above age 65 where the disabled respondents were more often single or widowed, separated, or divorced. Forty three per cent of disabled respondents lived alone compared with 30 per cent of the non-disabled respondents. The social class distribution is shown in Table 4.2, which indicates that there are consistently smaller proportions of disabled people in social classes I and II than there are for the control sample.

Table 4.1. *Proportion of disabled and non-disabled respondents by age and sex at first interview*

| | Disabled sample | | Non-disabled sample | | All respondents | |
Age	Men (%)	Women (%)	Men (%)	Women (%)	Disabled (%)	Non-disabled (%)
16–24	6	5	15	14	5	15
25–44	15	18	30	36	17	33
45–64	50	43	25	22	46	23
65–77	29	34	30	28	32	29
Total	100	100	100	100	100	100
N	395	492	146	201	887	347

There were no significant differences between disabled and control respondents in the proportions of persons who were white and non-white; overall 15 per cent of the sample were non-white, and this proportion decreased with age. Likewise, there was no significant difference between the two samples in place of birth: 24 per cent were born in Lambeth, 52 per cent elsewhere in the UK, 9 per cent in Europe, 9 per cent in the West Indies, and 5 per cent in Africa, the Far East, or the Indian subcontinent. These figures are similar to those for the Lambeth borough as a whole. Only 15 (2 per cent) of the disabled respondents lived in sheltered or warden-assisted accommodations.

Table 4.2. *Proportion of disabled and non-disabled respondents by household social class and age*

Social class	Age Category									
	16–24		24–45		45–64		65–77		All Ages	
	Disabled (%)	Control (%)	Disabled (%)	Control (%)	Disabled (%)	Control (%)	Disabled (%)	Control (%)	Disabled (%)	Control (%)
I and II	17	23	26	34	15	24	14	20	17	27
III Non-manual	19	19	15	28	24	18	21	17	21	18
III Manual	41	35	26	28	30	24	31	26	30	28
IV and V	23	23	33	18	31	34	34	37	32	27
Total	100	100	100	100	100	100	100	100	100	100
N	48	48	138	110	397	77	264	91	847	326

Number of missing observations = 61

Respondents lost to the study

While non-response is a problem with any survey, it can be particularly serious in longitudinal health surveys, especially if drop-out is related to major variables of interest. For example, less healthy people are more likely to die or to become institutionalized than are healthy individuals. Moreover, response rates at each stage are multiplicative; even an 80 per cent response rate on each of three follow-ups results in a group composed of little over 50 per cent of those originally sampled. In the Lambeth Health Survey a newsletter which reported the results of the survey to respondents was used to maintain respondent interest in the study and to ensure a good response. This was moderately successful in keeping the response rate for all respondents at each stage above 80 per cent.

In any study the respondents should be compared with the non-respondents as much as possible to explore the extent to which the results might be biased by the exclusion of non-respondents. The 380 (31 per cent) respondents who were lost to the study between the first interview and the final one were compared in terms of their characteristics with the 860 respondents who remained. Socio–demographic data and variables describing social and formal service support, number of medical conditions and symptoms, and disability scores were compared to see whether there were any statistically significant differences between the two groups (chi-squared tests for the discrete variables and univariate analyses of variance for the continuous ones). Separate analyses were performed for the disabled and control groups. There were only a few significant differences at the 5 per cent level. In the disabled sample, males were more likely not to respond than females. In the control sample there was a higher percentage of non-respondents among younger and single people. Twenty-two per cent of non-respondents were aged 16–24, as opposed to 11 per cent of respondents. Among single people 39 per cent did not respond, compared with 22 per cent of the rest of the sample. Here too, non-respondents tended to have fewer medical symptoms (mean of 1.3 as opposed to a mean of 1.9 for the respondents).

Non-response in the control sample might have been due to lack of interest in a study of disability. This suggestion is supported by the fact that, overall, the response rate in the control group was lower than in the disabled group. For the disabled sample it does not appear that those lost to follow-up were different from the final study group, but the same cannot be said for the control sample in which non-respondents tended to be younger and to have fewer medical symptoms.

In planning longitudinal studies it is important to minimize the time interval between initial screening and the first interview to avoid losing severely ill individuals. During the 6–9 months period between the screening study and the first interview in the Lambeth survey, 24 (2 per cent) of the potential disabled respondents and 1 of the potential control respondents died. The numbers of respondents who had entered institutions or had become too ill to take part in the study were 16 and 1, respectively. Thus, comparatively few individuals were lost in this manner. Between the first and third interview, 54 (6 per cent) of the disabled and 2 (2 per cent) of the control sample died. Twenty one (2 per cent) of the disabled also became too ill to be interviewed or had entered an institution.

Disability measurement in both samples

As described in the Chapter 3, the FLP was employed as the disability measure in the longitudinal study. For the remainder of this chapter, attention is focused on respondents aged 25–77, since only 5 per cent of the disabled sample were aged 16–24. To combine the latter group with the older respondents is inappropriate because of differences in type of impairments and level of social support, given that many younger respondents were living with their parents.

Ten per cent of the disabled sample had an FLP score of zero on first interview, and 32 per cent of the control group had a score greater than zero. Since the time interval between screening and the first interview was 6–12 months, some of this difference may be due to a change in disability status. As Table 4.3 shows, most of the control group had minor disabilities, with only 7 per cent having a score of 5 or more. The most frequent screening items endorsed by disabled persons who reported disablement at screening, but not at interview, were 'spells of giddiness and fits' (13 per cent), 'other recreational and pastime activity restrictions'

Table 4.3. *Overall disability level of disabled and non-disabled sample at first interview by age group*

Disability level on FLP	Disabled sample		Non-disabled sample	
	Aged 25–64 (%)	Aged 65–77 (%)	Aged 25–64 (%)	Aged 65–77 (%)
0	10.9	6.0	73.1	53.5
−5	29.2	19.2	23.4	33.3
−20	37.3	38.1	3.0	13.1
Over −20	22.6	36.7	0.5	0.0
N	558	281	197	99

(9 per cent), and 'weakness or paralysis of the arms or legs' (8 per cent).

Fig. 4.2 shows how the disabled and non-disabled of similar age and sex compared in terms of their scores on the 12 FLP categories at first interview. The disabled and non-disabled are most similar in the cateogries 'eating' and 'communication'. Among the disabled in both age groups, women tended to obtain higher scores than men except for the categories of 'social interaction' and 'alertness', and 'emotion' for the age group 25–64, where the two sexes were very similar. The profiles for men and women in the two groups are not similar. Most striking are the higher 'household management' and lower 'work' disability scores for women.

Measurement properties of the Functional Limitations Profile

Since the FLP was being applied for the first time in a household interview survey in England, the properties of the instrument were examined carefully (Charlton *et al.* 1983). Of particular interest was how well summary measures composed from FLP items would perform, compared with the use of the original 12 or more separate sub-scores. Global health status indicators enable cross-disease comparisons by reflecting outcomes on a set of common dimensions. The comparison process becomes increasingly difficult, however, as the number of indicators used increases. One

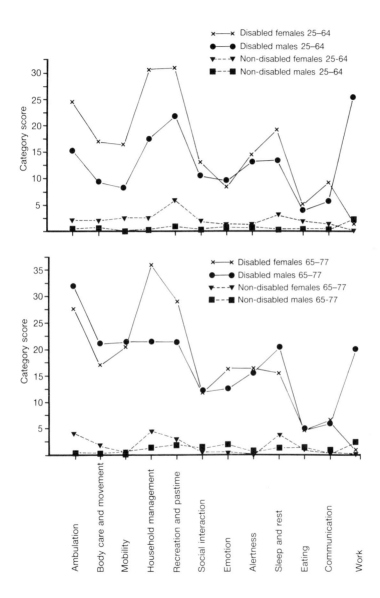

Fig. 4.2. Comparison of Functional Limitations Profile category scores of disabled and non-disabled samples by age and sex.

objective in examining the responses to the FLP items was to determine the minimum number of scores necessary to describe disability in community surveys.

Using multidimensional scaling and cluster analysis on both cross-sectional and longitudinal data, a series of 5 global measures were derived from the 136 FLP items. These measures were: (1) a psychosocial score comprising emotion, alertness, sleep and rest, and recreation; (2) a physical score comprising walking, confinement, movement, self-care, mobility, and household management; (3) eating; (4) communication; and (5) work. Fig. 4.3 shows a graphic representation of the global measures and the similarities between component parts. In this type of representation, the distances between pairs of points are directly related to the

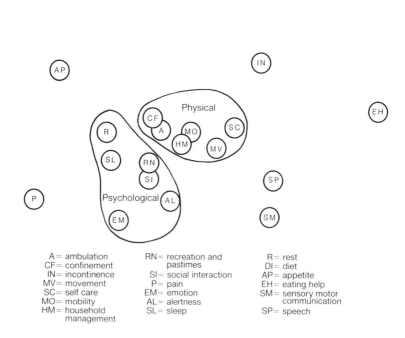

A = ambulation	RN = recreation and pastimes	R = rest
CF = confinement		DI = diet
IN = incontinence	SI = social interaction	AP = appetite
MV = movement	P = pain	EH = eating help
SC = self care	EM = emotion	SM = sensory motor communication
MO = mobility	AL = alertness	
HM = household management	SL = sleep	SP = speech

Fig. 4.3. Association between category scores for disabled respondents aged 25–77 years at first interview.

strength of the association between the items. The aim is to group similar items close together.

Evaluation of the FLP as a global measure of health status

The repeatability of the global measures and individual items over 2 days was tested on a small sample of 30 disabled patients attending a health clinic. Although changes in the global scores were generally smaller than those in the individual category scores, there were individual category scores, such as those for 'walking', which changed the least. The magnitude of the changes ranged from −2.68 to 6.5. The repeatability of individual items varied from 22 per cent to 100 per cent, which suggests that items should not be used independently.

The global measures were more sensitive in identifying disabled respondents than were the individual categories. A relatively high proportion of respondents who were identified by the global measures 'physical' and 'psychosocial' disability were missed by individual category scores. 'Walking' and 'household management' were areas in which a relatively large number of people with 'physical' disability were identified (89 per cent and 84 per cent, respectively).

Although other factors also are important, disability should be of some value in discriminating between people who do and do not make use of services. Category scores and global measures were compared for their ability to discriminate between people who had and had not registered their disability with the local authority to receive services, and those who had and had not seen their doctor in the previous 2 weeks. The global and category disability scores were significantly related to service use. Fig. 4.4 shows, for the total FLP score, the proportions of respondents with different FLP scores who had used home-help services in the previous 14 days and were registered as disabled.

The false-positive and false-negative rates for classifying individuals as users or non-users were high, however. When used in conjunction with 'work', 'communication' and 'eating', the two global measures of 'physical' and 'psychosocial' disability performed approximately as well as the full set of 12 category measures. All category scores and the global health status

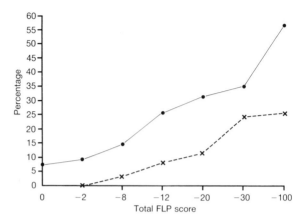

Fig. 4.4. Proportion of disabled patients in Functional Limitations Profile grade who were registered as disabled (bottom line) and had seen home help in the previous 14 days (top line).

measures were equally bad predictors of individual service use. This lack of discrimination could be due to a lack of measurement sensitivity in the FLP, which combines several activities that may be performed at different levels of function within the same question (Jette 1980). At the same time, it could be due to a misfit between function status and service use, since it is known that many other factors besides health status influence the use of service.

Thus, although and advantages of greater repeatability and precision, which are claimed for global health status measures, could not be demonstrated, the 5 global dimensions (physical, psychosocial, communication, eating, and work) provide a smaller number of scores with which to work and thus aid description. The instrument still comprises 136 statements, but the 5 scores provide a basis for reducing this number. Since the repeatability of certain items is low, those items should not be used individually. The repeatability of measures combining several items is higher, and the 2 global measures, especially physical disability, were found to have repeatability and standard errors that are generally better than those of .the individual category scores, although some category scores were just as good in this respect.

Statistical properties of disability measures

For most of the individuals surveyed in a community sample the category scores are the weighted sums of relatively few items, and therefore they take a limited number of discrete values. Combining similar categories into larger, global measures should improve statistical properties and simplify the description and analysis of disability in populations, provided that the measures remain meaningful. Fig. 4.5 shows the distributions of one of the category scores (mobility), and one of the global measures (physical disability). The global measure has a smoother distribution, although the distribution is still J-shaped. Fig. 4.6 shows the distribution of change in scores for physical disability over a 1-year period, which more closely approximates a normal distribution. The distribution of any disability measure will have to be taken into account in its analysis.

One part of the longitudinal study was an experiment to investigate the effects that different interviewers might have on the results (Wiggins 1984). It is well-known that interviewers can

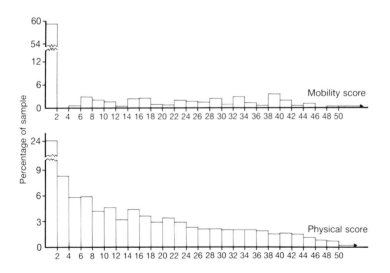

Fig. 4.5. Distribution of mobility (category) and physical (global) disability scores at first interview.

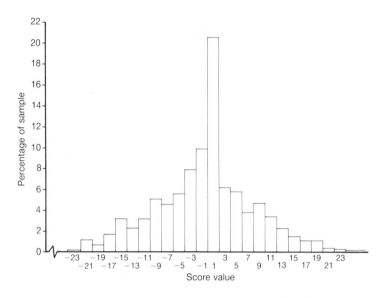

Fig. 4.6. Distribution of change in physical score over a year.

influence the answers to survey questions, but little work has been done on health status or disability measures. Wards in the central part of the Borough of Lambeth were selected for the experiment. The respondents were systematically divided into 12 assignments, and interviews were allocated randomly to the 12 interviewers. In the first year of the study, interviewer effects accounted for 5 per cent or more of the total variation in a fifth of the FLP items and 10 per cent or more for 4 (3 per cent) of the items. Negligible interviewer effects were found for basic socio–demographic variables. These results are similar to those obtained in an interviewer variability study conducted by Collins (1978) on a sample of disabled people in Southampton. The results for the second interview in the Lambeth survey produced a similar distribution, although the estimated effects for individual items were not necessarily the same.

Interviewer effects for the 12 category scores tended to be smaller, ranging from 0 to 9 per cent, where 'emotion', 'recreation', and 'sleep and rest' were most affected (9 per cent, 6 per cent and 5 per cent, respectively, at first interview, and 3 per cent, 3 per cent, and 1 per cent at second interview). Thus when using global scores, as has been the case with most analyses in this study, it seems that interviewer effects on the results are likely to be small, although no precise estimates have been made concerning the magnitude of such effects.

Measuring changes in disability

As shown previously, disability scores can vary considerably over a short period of time and from one year to the next. From an epidemiological point of view it is interesting to be able to predict those people who are likely to deteriorate steadily and those who are likely to improve. Since we had three observations on each individual in our study, it is possible to use the middle observation to define whether any trend is consistent. There are a number of ways to do this, and one of the least complicated methods, involving the categorization of respondents into groups, was chosen for this study. The FLP is intended to be an equal-interval scale, that is, differences of the same magnitude between any pair of values are of equal importance. From our experience of the FLP, based on comparisons between disabled and non-disabled people and items endorsed at various FLP levels, a change of magnitude of 5 units or more appears to be a meaningful one. This also is the finding of Deyo *et al.* (1982). Using data on disability level from all three phases of the study, respondents were categorized into the following groups on the basis of their physical, psychosocial, and category scores:

1. Steady deteriorators whose disability scores *increased* by 5 units or more between first and third interviews, while the second interview score was not more than 5 units *below* the first interview value.
2. Steady improvers whose disability scores *decreased* by 5 units or more between first and third interviews, while the second interview score was not more than 5 units *above* the first interview value.
3. Negligible changers whose scores on the second and third interviews were within 5 units of the initial score.
4. Ambiguous changers who do not fit into the above categories since their scores on the first and third interviews increased or decreased by 5 units, but their second interview scores were

more than 5 units in the opposite direction to the change between first and third interviews.

Once such change categories were defined, simple comparisons could be made in tabular form. If the joint effects of several variables are to be considered simultaneously, the comparisons between pairs of change groups, for example between 'steady deteriorators' and 'no change', can be made using logistic regression (Cox 1971). If more than two change groups are to be modelled simultaneously, log-linear modelling can be employed, (Nelder 1974, Goodman 1973). Both types of analysis can easily be accomplished in computer packages such as GLIM. Some approaches, which were not used in this study, include Goldstein's (1979) use of preceding observations to predict present ones, as in his study to predict the reading age of schoolchildren. Here he used previous reading ages and previous social classes. In models involving even two or three measurements taken at various times, the analysis can become quite complicated when more than two time periods are involved. Thus, the change between second and third interviews could be predicted on the basis of the first and second interviews responses, but the possibilities are numerous. When multiple dependent variables are involved, path analysis can be employed (see Johnston 1972), while more complex methods have been developed by Jöreskog (1977), which Goldstein suggests should be used only with caution, since it is seldom possible to test whether the assumptions on which these models are based are valid.

Two-year disability changes in Lambeth

Using the four categories of change in disability status previously described, Table 4.4 shows the percentages of respondents in the disabled and non-disabled samples who had disability levels that deteriorated, improved, stayed constant, or fluctuated. Less than 6 per cent of the control sample were steady deteriorators, and less than 6 per cent of them were steady improvers, for both the physical or psychosocial scores. Disabled respondents classified according to the same categories were similar on demographic characteristics such as age, sex, housing tenure, household composition, and nature of the medical condition interfering most with daily activities. Of the steady deteriorators, 42 per cent were aged 65–77, 62 per cent were female, 75 per cent lived with others, and 63 per cent had four or more medical conditions. Table 4.5 shows the joint distribution of respondents between the four categories of physical and psychosocial changes for the disabled sample. Respondents did not necessarily change in the same direction or to the same extent on both measures, and the change categories are identical for only 51 per cent of the sample. Most of the changes occurred in those aged 45–77. In the younger age group only 12 of the 103 disabled deteriorated and 16 improved.

Tables 4.6 and 4.7 show the relationship between the change in physical and psychosocial disability score between the first and third interviews and the initial level of disability at the first interview. Deterioration and improvement in physical disability are highly associated with initial level of disability. To a certain extent this is inevitable, since for a bedridden person there is less scope for further deterioration and more scope for improvement than there is for a less disabled individual. Of those with the greatest disability level 7 per cent detriorated, 37 per cent improved, and 30 per cent fluctuated, while for those with moderate or minor disability the comparable figures were 34, 14, and 19 per cent. This finding is consistent with regression toward the mean, but it is unlikely to be the entire explanation since the moderate disability group, not the low disability group, was the group most at risk of deterioration. There also was a strong

Table 4.4. *Proportion of disabled and non-disabled sample falling into each change category between first and third interviews*

Category	Disabled sample		Control sample	
	Physical score	Psychosocial score	Physical score	Psychosocial score
Steady deteriorators	23.8	23.7	4.9	5.4
Steady improvers	19.7	27.5	3.6	5.8
Negligible changers	35.2	30.2	88.4	83.9
Ambiguous changers	21.3	18.6	3.1	4.9
N	630		224	

Table 4.5. *Number of disabled persons in the physical and psychosocial change categories*

| | | Psychosocial score | | | | |
		Steady deteriorators	Steady improvers	Negligible change	Ambiguous	Total
Physical score	Steady deteriorators	80	16	28	26	150
	Steady improvers	10	75	24	15	124
	Negligible change	28	34	125	35	222
	Ambiguous	31	48	14	41	134
	N	149	173	191	117	630

Table 4.6. *Change in physical disability level between first and third interviews**

Initial disability level		Change Category			
		Deteriorators %	Improvers %	Stable %	Ambiguous %
Physical	0–8	21	1	42	7
disability	9–20	50	31	31	38
score at	›20	29	68	27	55
1st					
interview					
N		115	105	109	104

*Excludes under 45-year-olds and those scoring zero on FLP

Table 4.7. *Change in psychosocial disability level between first and third interviews**

Initial disability level		Change Category			
		Deteriorators %	Improvers %	Stable %	Ambiguous %
Psychosocial	0–8	38	0	51	7
disability	9–20	49	38	39	47
score at	›20	13	62	10	46
1st					
interview					
N psychosocial		114	130	95	94

*Excludes under 45-year-olds and those scoring zero on FLP

association between change in psychosocial disability and initial level of disability. Unlike the case of physical disability, the group most likely to deteriorate was the one with the lowest initial levels, and the proportion deteriorating decreased with increasing initial level. Conversely, people with greater disability were most likely

80   *Measuring disability in a longitudinal survey*

to improve. There may be greater regression toward the mean with psychosocial disability than with physical disability, but other explanations are possible.

References

Charlton, J. R. H., Patrick, D. L., and Peach, H. (1983). Use of multivariate measures of disability in health surveys. *Journal of Epidemiology and Community Health* **37**, 296–304.
Collins, M. (1978). *Interviewer variability: North Yorkshire Experiment.* Methodological Working Paper No. 13. London: Social and Community Planning Research.
Cox, D. (1971). *The analysis of binary data* Methuen, London.
Deyo, R. A., Inui, T. S., and Leininger, J. D. *et al.* (1982). Physical and psychosocial function in rheumatoid arthritis. *Archives Internal Medicine* **142**, 879–82.
Goldstein, H. (1979) *The design and analysis of longitudinal studies: their role in the measurement of change.* Academic Press, London.
Goodman, L. A. (1973). The analysis of multidimensional contingency tables when some variables are posterior to others: a modified path analysis approach. *Biometrika* **60**, 1179–259.
Jette, A. M. (1980). Health status indicators: their utility in chronic disease evaluation research. *Journal of Chronic Diseases* **33**, 567–79.
Johnston, J. (1972). *Econometric methods* (2nd edn.) McGraw-Hill, New York.
Jöreskog, K. G. (1977). Statistical models and methods for analysis of longitudinal data. In *Latent variables in socio-economic models.* (ed D. V. Aigner and A. S. Goldberger) Elsevier North Holland, Amsterdam.
Nelder, J. A. (1974). Log-linear models for contingency tables: a generalization of classical least squares. *Applied Statistics* **23**, 323–29.
Ritchie, J. and Patrick, D. (forthcoming). *The Lambeth Health Survey: methodological report.* London: Social and Community Planning Research.
Wiggins, R. D. (1984). *A study of interviewer effects in a longitudinal survey of the physically handicapped* ESRC (end of grant report).

5

Impairment and disability

HEDLEY PEACH

The ICIDH views disability as the result of impairment and impairment as the result of disease or disorder, as shown in Fig. 1.1. This scheme implies that the level of disability in a community may be reduced by preventing the medical conditions and impairments that lead to disability. Thus the level of disability in a community could be reduced by the primary and secondary prevention of disease (primary prevention of disability) or the effective treatment of disabling symptoms (secondary prevention of disability). The first step is to discern which ailments and untreated symptoms contribute the most to the level of disability and which activities are most restricted.

The 9 divisions of impairment outlined by the ICIDH in Table 5.1 were used to devise the Lambeth questionnaire. We excluded from the list of impairments physical signs and all items that were applicable only to children and to the mentally handicapped, since these groups were not included in the survey. Items that were uncommon among disabled adults and sexual impairments were also left out. The repeatability of the medical questionnaire was tested over 2 days and 2 weeks among hospital out-patients. The

Table 5.1. *Main divisions in the classification of impairments*

1.	Intellectual
2.	Other psychological
3.	Language
4.	Aural
5.	Ocular
6.	Visceral
7.	Skeletal
8.	Disfiguring
9.	Generalized, sensory, and other

validity of patient's statements concerning their medical conditions, the symptoms they claimed to have reported to their doctors, and the medications they said that they were taking were confirmed in interviews with the clinic doctors. The repeatability of the medical questionnaire was satisfactory (at least 80 per cent over 2 weeks for each item), and there was close agreement between statements made by the patients and clinic doctors (at least 80 per cent for each item).

Disease and disability

Table 5.2 lists the diseases and disorders that Lambeth respondents said interfered with their daily activities the most. A quarter or a fifth of the respondents were unable to identify a 'main' debilitating disease or disorder. The remainder gave a wide variety of main medical problems as indicated by the large number of diseases and disorders mentioned by less than 1 per cent of the respondents in all three age groups. Sciatica or lumbago was most

Table 5.2. *Diseases and disorders that disabled respondents said most interfered with their daily activities*

Disease or disorder	Per cent of respondents by age group		
	25–44	45–64	65–75
Arthritis	6	12	31
Sciatica/lumbago	12	6	4
Bronchitis	2	4	6
Asthma	4	4	1
Heart disease	1	4	4
High blood-pressure	4	3	3
Depression	5	4	2
Hay fever	1	0	0
Epilepsy	3	2	1
Other*	37	41	28
None in particular	25	20	20
N	121	349	232

*Includes those diseases and disorders mentioned by less than 1 per cent of the respondents in all three age groups.

frequently mentioned by respondents aged 25 to 44. Respondents who were middle-aged (aged 45 to 64) and elderly (aged 65 to 75) said arthritis was the main disabling condition. Respondents under the age of 65 were less likely than the elderly to identify a main disease or disorder and more likely to list a wider variety of ailments that hindered their daily activities.

The OPCS National Survey found that arthritis, blindness, stroke, coronary heart disease, and bronchitis were the diseases and disorders most frequently mentioned by respondents as the main cause of their disabilities (Harris 1971). Similarly, Warren (1974) found that the most common causes of disability in his survey of Canterbury households were arthritis, rheumatism, stroke, and heart disease, although mental disorders were also important. Bennett and Garrad (1970) found that respiratory, arthritic, cardiovascular, and cerebrovascular diseases were the most frequently mentioned primary diagnoses among their random sample of disabled people living in North Lambeth. The chief diseases and disorders found in these surveys are similar to those indicated by the disabled respondents in Lambeth, even though the surveys were conducted on different samples, at different times, and with different definitions of disability.

The main drawback of asking respondents which disease or disorder interferes with their lives the most is that this information does not tell us how the disease or disorder interferes. To obtain such information, the researchers compared the disability profiles of respondents with the different diseases or disorders mentioned by the respondents.

Figure 5.1 shows the disability or FLPs of three conditions that respondents said interfered with their daily activities the most: hypertension, bronchitis, and arthritis. The activities in which respondents were least restricted were the same for all three conditions, namely eating and drinking, and communication, which includes talking and writing. For all three ailments, respondents were very restricted in household management, recreation and pastimes, and ambulation, which includes walking and climbing stairs. Respondents who said arthritis interfered with their daily activities the most were more restricted in housework, getting around inside and outside the house, and body care and movement of limbs than were respondents who said hypertension or bronchitis interfered the most. Respondents who said their

Category

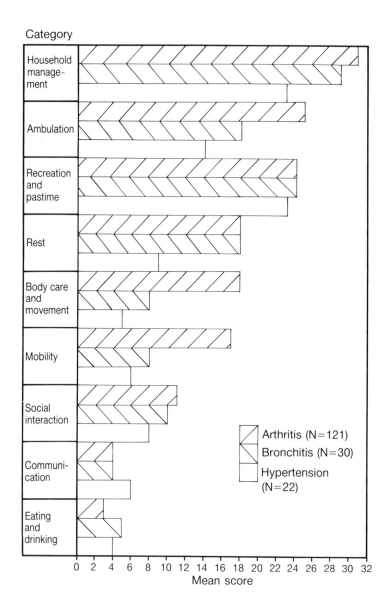

Fig. 5.1. Average Functional Limitations Profile category scores of respondents with different disabling conditions.

main problem was hypertension were the least restricted in most activities.

Although we were able to establish whether the FLP of respondents with particular main diseases differed from one another, it was impossible to attribute these differences to the main disease alone, because respondents reported many other diseases as well. Disabled respondents had an average of three medical conditions each, with a total range of 1 to 12 conditions.

Each disease or disorder was cited by a relatively small number of respondents as the most interfering, compared with the number of respondents who reported having the disease or disorder. For

Table 5.3. *Disease and disorders reported by respondents at second interview by age group and sex*

Disease or disorder	Men			Women		
	25–44 (%)	45–64 (%)	65–75 (%)	25–44 (%)	45–64 (%)	65–75 (%)
Bronchitis	16	27	37	18	21	29
Arthritis	22	44	41	37	55	75
Sciatica	33	34	31	50	41	45
Skin trouble	21	14	13	15	11	12
Asthma				18	8	5
Hayfever	22	12	8	24	11	8
Stomach ulcers	9	10	6			
Haemorrhoids	7	17	10	15	13	11
Hypertension	7	21	21	10	23	31
Heart trouble	5	25	30	5	19	22
Foot trouble	21	16	17	20	33	31
Varicose veins	5	14	17	16	21	22
Depression	30	23	20	33	42	35
Diabetes				4	6	11
Cataracts	4	4	13	1	4	11
Stroke	0	6	13			
Prostate trouble	4	7	14			
N	76	186	138	45	163	94

Excludes diseases and disorders reported by less than 10 per cent of respondents in all three age groups example, only 10 to 30 per cent of respondents with arthritis, bronchitis, and hypertension indicated that these diseases hindered their daily activities the most.

Among middle-aged and elderly men the most frequently reported conditions were arthritis, bronchitis, sciatica, heart disease, hypertension, and depression (Table 5.3). Among younger men the most frequently reported medical problems were the same except that hay fever, skin trouble, and foot trouble replaced heart disease and hypertension.

Among middle-aged and elderly women the most frequently reported diseases and disorders were the same as those reported by the men with the addition of foot trouble. These ailments were also most frequently reported by younger women, but hay fever replaced foot trouble, bronchitis, heart trouble, and hypertension. As expected, the reporting of most chronic conditions increased with age. The only ones that decreased with age were hay fever, skin trouble, asthma, and depression in men, but not in women.

Not all of the disease and disorders reported in a community survey can be expected to be equally disabling. Harris (1971) found that the conditions with the highest proportion of very severely handicapped people were multiple sclerosis, Parkinson's disease, stroke, paraplegia/hemiplegia, cerebral palsy, and arthritis. Those least likely to handicap people as far as self-care was concerned were sciatica, skin disease, and epilepsy. Although people suffering from multiple sclerosis, Parkinson's disease, or stroke were likely to be very severely or severely handicapped rather than merely impaired, the total number of handicapped people suffering from such incapacitating diseases were relatively small in the national OPCS survey. This finding indicates that arthritis is responsible for severely handicapping most impaired people. Arthritis and rheumatism are also the leading causes of disability in the US (DeJong and Lifchez 1983).

To discover which medical conditions reported by disabled people in Lambeth contributed the most to the overall level of disability in the borough, the researchers used the statistical technique of multiple regression. Table 5.4 shows the result of regressing each of 9 category scores of the FLP on all the diseases and disorders reported by the disabled in Lambeth. With the exception of eating and drinking, the conditions significantly associated with a category score explained about 20 to 30 per cent

Table 5.4. *Diseases and disorders associated with different categories on the Functional Limitations Profile*

Disease or disorder	Communication	Eating and drinking	Body care and movement of limbs	Ambulation	Mobility	Household management	Rest	Recreation and pastime	Social interaction
Depression	0.83	0.47	0.07	0.95	1.85	1.11	1.99	1.60	0.07
Stroke	1.71	0.69	0.07	1.88	2.07	1.85	1.16	2.07	0.07
Arthritis			0.07	0.60	0.52	1.46			0.07
Sciatica			0.06						0.06
Foot trouble				0.56	0.68		0.63	0.76	0.06
Hypertension		0.60					0.83	1.22	
Heart trouble		0.46					0.69	0.88	
Bronchitis				0.51					
Asthma								1.09	
Diabetes		1.46							
Cataracts	1.68								
Haemorrhoids		0.46						0.92	

N = 702
Only statistically significant regression coefficients are shown.

of the variance in disability. Depression and stroke were associated with restriction in all activities. Arthritis was associated mainly with physical disability: body care and movement of limbs, walking and climbing stairs, getting around inside and outside the house. Sciatica or lumbago and hypertension were associated mainly with social disability: resting during the day, recreation and pastime, and (in the case of sciatica only) social interaction with family and friends.

Harris (1971) found that stroke and arthritis were associated with appreciable disability, or worse, in a large percentage of respondents with these conditions. However, she found that sciatica was associated with appreciable disability only in a very small percentage of respondents suffering from it. As discussed in Chapter 2, the discrepancy between our prevalence estimate and that of Harris can be explained by the definition of disability used in the national OPCS survey, which included only self-care activities and ignored the psychosocial aspects of disability.

The association between the various medical conditions and the FLP category scores is likely to be direct and causal, except in the case of depression where disability is just as likely to lead to depression as result from it. The association between psychosocial disability and hypertension is an interesting one. Haynes *et al.* (1978) found that absenteeism from work increased after the detection and labelling of hypertensive employees, although Alderman and Davies (1976) found the opposite effect.

Symptoms and disability

In addition to reporting medical diagnoses, respondents in the Lambeth survey reported their symptoms as shown in Table 5.5. Among men aged 25 to 44, pain or stiffness in the back or joints, difficulty sleeping, and headaches were the most frequently reported symptoms. The symptoms most frequently reported by middle-aged men included all of those as well as shortness of breath, tiredness, paralysis, weakness or numbness of limbs, and constipation. Among the symptoms reported by elderly men, it was difficult to select any that were reported more frequently than others except for shortness of breath, pain and stiffness in joints, and productive cough.

Headaches and being overweight were the symptoms reported

Table 5.5. *Symptoms reported by respondents at the second interview by age group and sex*

	Men			Women		
Symptom	25–44 (%)	45–64 (%)	65–75 (%)	25–44 (%)	45–64 (%)	65–75 (%)
Pain in joints	37	38	37	41	57	57
Difficulty sleeping	18	31	25	39	41	49
Stiffness in joints	28	36	30	30	36	40
Tiredness or weakness	33	27	26	37	44	40
Pain or stiffness in back	55	25	21	35	36	38
Shortness of breath hurrying on level ground or slight hill	16	33	45	35	42	35
Swelling of feet or ankles	0	17	18	26	38	33
Difficulty keeping balance	18	19	25	16	29	32
Headaches	36	29	19	65	47	30
Difficulty seeing	12	16	22	16	23	28
Depression	22	16	18	22	32	27
Giddiness	14	14	21	22	25	23
Shortness of breath walking with people of own age	3	24	29	12	26	28
Overweight	22	27	12	46	33	22
Calf pain	14	13	16	14	23	22
Feeling hot and shaky	12	12	11	22	38	20
Constipation	0	11	11	7	11	19
Trouble hearing	12	12	19	10	17	18
Trouble learning, remembering, or thinking clearly	0	19	17	12	14	17
Pain in eyes	8	6	14	15	14	17
Ringing in ears	9	15	21	12	14	16
Limbs paralysed, weak, or numb	22	25	26	15	25	16
Frequency of urination	3	9	18	8	16	14
Stomach pains	0	14	13	26	15	13
Dry cough or sore throat	22	16	22	19	19	12
Cough with phlegm	14	22	36	15	21	11
Chest pain	20	14	20	18	18	11
Loss of appetite	0	12	11	10	12	10
Shortness of breath washing or dressing	0	13	19			
Shortness of breath sitting quietly	16	6	11			
N	76	186	138	45	163	94

Excludes symptoms reported by less than 10 per cent of respondents in all three age groups

Table 5.6. *Symptoms associated with different categories of the Functional Limitations Profile*

Symptom	Communication	Eating and drinking	Body care and movement of limbs	Ambulation	Mobility	Household management	Rest	Recreation and pastime	Social interaction
Difficulty getting to sleep or staying asleep			0.07	0.63	0.65	0.90	1.68	0.99	0.70
Difficulty keeping balance on feet			0.14	1.67	0.99	1.48	0.76	1.36	0.76
General tiredness or weakness					0.62	0.59	1.32	1.16	0.81
Trouble learning remembering or thinking clearly	2.21					0.73	0.75	1.25	0.89
Limbs paralysed deformed, missing, or broken	1.28	1.0	1.0	0.89	1.25	1.36	1.10	1.07	0.83
Pain or stiffness in joints or back			0.05	0.57	0.83	1.01	1.06	0.99	0.75
Swelling of feet or ankles				1.09	0.63		1.02	0.74	0.51
Shortness of breath		0.37		0.51				0.45	
Trouble seeing, hearing, or talking	1.91								
Constipation		1.57						0.75	
Loss of appetite or weight		1.24							
Pain in stomach								0.96	
Pain in calves								5.43	
Frequency or incontinence of urine			0.09	0.69	0.98		0.74	0.91	0.72

N = 702
Only statistically significant regression coefficients are shown

most frequently by women aged 25 to 44. Other symptoms often reported in this age group included all those reported by men the same age as well as tiredness and shortness of breath. Among middle-aged women the most frequently reported symptoms included all those reported by younger women plus swelling of feet or ankles; spells of feeling upset, depressed, or crying; spells of feeling hot, nervous, or shaky; and difficulty in keeping balance. As with the elderly men, it was difficult to select any symptoms that were reported more frequently than others for elderly women except for pain in joints and difficulty sleeping.

To find out which symptoms contributed the most to the overall level of disability, the 9 FLP category scores were regressed on all the reported symptoms. Table 5.6 identifies the symptoms that are significantly associated with each FLP score. With the exception of the communication and eating and drinking categories, the symptoms associated with each of the categories explained between 30 and 40 per cent of the variance.

Few studies have tried to relate symptoms with disability. Morrell and Wale (1976) asked a random sample of women aged 20 to 44, who were registered with a general practice, to keep a health diary for 28 days, recording any symptoms of illness they perceived and their responses to them, which included activity restrictions and lying down. 'Changes in energy or tiredness' were associated with disability in 54 per cent of symptom days, disturbance of menstruation and cough in 46 per cent, and abdominal pain, cold, and backache in about 40 per cent. The sample and method of recording disability in this study were entirely different from those of the Lambeth study, but in both studies tiredness, back pain, and emotional symptoms were associated with disability.

Untreated symptoms among the disabled

Several studies have shown that people obtain treatment from their general practitioner or a hospital for only a small proportion of their symptoms. The survey of sickness (Stocks 1949) found that less than a quarter of those complaining of illness had seen a doctor about it. This proportion was confirmed by a survey in Bermondsey and Southwark (Wadsworth *et al.* 1971). Dunnell and Cartwright (1972) provided further evidence of a large 'iceberg' of illness in the general population at any one time that is not reported to the medical profession. Although 91 per cent of the adults in Dunnell and Cartwright's study reported having symptoms during the 2 weeks before interview, only 17 per cent had consulted a doctor during that time and 28 per cent of the adults said that they had not consulted their general practitioner at all during the previous 12-month period. Therefore, it is likely that a large proportion of the Lambeth respondents who had symptoms that were significantly associated with disability had not reported the symptoms to their doctors.

The fact that most people do not report their symptoms to a doctor does not mean that those symptoms are untreated. Dunnell and Cartwright (1972) found that 55 per cent of their adult respondents said they had taken or used some medicine during the 24 hours before interview, although only 16 per cent had consulted a doctor. Other studies have also found that self-medication was more common than professional treatment. Dunnell and Cartwright found that for every prescribed item taken in a 2-week period there were two non-prescribed items. In accordance with these findings, the symptoms reported by the disabled persons in Lambeth fall into one of three groups: those that have been reported to a doctor, those that have not been reported to a doctor but are being treated by the respondents themselves, and those that have not been reported to a doctor or treated by the respondents.

If unreported and untreated symptoms are associated with disability, it may be possible to reduce the level of disability by encouraging people to report their symptoms and get them treated. For example, if difficulty sleeping interfered significantly with a patient's activities, the general practitioner might determine both the cause and possible effective treatments for the patient's sleep problem. Not all symptoms can be treated effectively, however. Still, unless patients with disabling symptoms bring them to the attention of the medical profession, patients who can be helped will go untreated.

There were many symptoms that Lambeth respondents had not reported to their doctors and were not being treated (Table 5.7). The number of different symptoms as well as the frequency of individual unreported and untreated symptoms were greater among women than men. Symptom by symptom, the frequency

Table 5.7. *Symptoms that respondents had not reported to doctors and were untreated*

Symptom	Men			Women		
	25–44 (%)	45–64 (%)	65–75 (%)	25–44 (%)	45–64 (%)	65–75 (%)
Difficulty sleeping	9	11	11	16	16	16
General tiredness or weakness	18	6	10	15	19	16
Spells of being upset, dpressed, or crying	14	7	7	20	14	14
Spells of giddiness	5	4	10			
Dry cough or sore throat				19	16	14
Trouble learning remembering, or thinking clearly				3	11	14
Swelling of feet or ankles				7	14	12
Overweight		13	5	23	14	12
Ringing in ears				8	9	11
Difficulty seeing				5	8	10
Pain in joints				8	17	10
Headaches				15	12	8
Spells of feeling hot, nervous, or shaky				12	18	6
Pain in eye				10	5	5
Loss of appetite	7	12	4			
Pain or stiffness in back				11	7	3
N	76	187	138	45	164	94

Excludes symptoms reported by less than 10 per cent of men or women in all three age groups.

of unreported, untreated symptoms was similar among middle-aged and elderly women. Clear age trends were evident for only four symptoms, three of which—spells of being upset, depressed, or crying; overweight; and headaches—decreased with age, whereas trouble learning, remembering, or thinking clearly increased with age.

Surveys of people over the age of 75 who live at home have drawn attention to the frequency of untreated symptoms that very

Table 5.8. *Symptoms that had been reported to a doctor but were untreated*

Symptom	Men			Women		
	25–44 (%)	45–64 (%)	65–75 (%)	25–44 (%)	45–64 (%)	65–75 (%)
Pain in joints	9	10	16	22	10	11
Difficulty keeping balance on feet	9	7	11	7	7	11
Limbs paralysed, weak, or numb	11	11	10			
General tiredness or weakness	5	10	9	18	13	17
Stiffness in joints	7	12	9	14	7	8
Overweight	14	13	7	16	15	1
Trouble seeing				5	4	12
Difficulty sleeping				4	6	10
Swelling of feet or ankles				11	10	9
Spells of giddiness				8	10	8
Pain or stiffness in back				16	7	8
Spells of feeling hot, nervous, or shaky				3	10	3
N	76	187	138	45	164	94

Excludes symptoms reported by less than 10 per cent of men or women in all three age groups.

elderly people have not reported to their general practitioners (Williamson *et al.* 1964). The frequency of unreported and untreated symptoms in Lambeth among middle-aged and elderly people suggest that these symptoms should receive as much consideration in a study of people between the ages of 25 and 75 as in a study of the very elderly.

Even when respondents reported their symptoms to physicians, not all symptoms were treated. In Lambeth, the percentage of untreated, although reported, symptoms was greater among women than men (Table 5.8). In most cases, the frequency of such symptoms was similar for each age group, suggesting that this category of symptoms is as important for younger disabled people as for the disabled elderly. Moreover, the number of reported but untreated symptoms was so similar to the number of unreported symptoms that equal attention should be given to both categories.

Contribution of untreated symptoms of disability

To find out the extent to which untreated symptoms affect the overall level of disability in Lambeth, disability was regressed on symptoms, which were first coded as reported or not reported to a doctor, then as treated or untreated. Although unreported and/or untreated symptoms were common, regression analysis showed that after taking reported and treated symptoms into account, only three untreated symptoms and four unreported symptoms were associated with disability. The three untreated symptoms were constipation, spells of giddiness, and shortness of breath. The four unreported symptoms were spells of feeling hot, nervous, or shaky; diarrhoea and/or vomiting; shortness of breath; and spells of giddiness. These symptoms were associated with disability for only one or two activities.

It was surprising to find so few unreported and untreated symptoms associated with disability, in view of the frequency with which unreported symptoms occurred and with which symptoms were reported but not treated. It appears that the symptoms that contributed the most to the level of disability in Lambeth had in fact been reported to a doctor and were being treated. Because the result was so unexpected, the severity of disability among disabled people with unreported and untreated symptoms was compared with that of disabled people who had reported and were being treated for those symptoms. If the result held, the former group should be less severely disabled than the latter. In fact, for all four of the unreported symptoms and all three of the untreated symptoms, except spells of giddiness, and extent of restriction in one or more activities best determined whether respondents reported the symptom and whether they were being treated. Factors taken into account were age, sex, social class, marital status, and ethnic origin.

A large number of factors have been said to determine whether a person takes a symptom to his or her general practitioner, including age, sex, marital status, occupation, absence of basic housing amenities, difficulties in running a household, brevity of stay in the house or neighbourhood, and lack of attachment to the neighbourhood. This list has been derived from many studies, each of which examined only a few factors at a time. In the case of psychological problems, Wadsworth *et al.* (1971) found that the number of medical complaints, which represented health status, was the best discriminator between those who did and did not report symptoms to a doctor. This finding is in agreement with the Lambeth survey, which found that the extent of restriction in one or more daily activities was the best discriminator between respondents who reported spells of being upset, being depressed, or crying. In a case-control study of adults aged 16 to 75 in a general practice, Ingham and Miller (1979) showed that for 5 symptoms (backache, tiredness, anxiety, depression, and irritability) the amount of distress the symptoms caused rather than the frequency or duration of the symptoms determined whether the symptoms were reported to the general practitioner. In the US financial constraints influence a person's decision to seek medical care. Therefore, findings from American studies on reporting of symptoms to doctors may not be applicable to the UK. Nevertheless, using univariate analysis Chen and Buck (1981) found, in the US, that self-assessment of health and age, but not ethnicity and sex, were significantly associated with whether subjects with seven symptoms (leg cramps, headaches, tiredness, pain or stiffness in joints, heart pain, back trouble, and shortness of breath) brought them to medical attention.

Primary and secondary prevention in reducing disability among adults.

Bronchitis, which is potentially preventable by reducing cigarette smoking, was associated with disability in only one activity: walking and climbing stairs. Depression, stroke, arthritis, sciatica, foot trouble, and hypertension were all associated with disability in several activities, but the only condition for which there appears to be a simple and effective method of prevention is stroke. In Britain, as in the US, the number of deaths due to stroke has dropped, particularly those caused by intracerebral haemorrhage. However, the extent to which this problem can be alleviated by treating hypertension is still unclear. In the past decade there has been a shift in the emphasis of treating raised blood-pressure only for severe and/or symptomatic hypertension to treating it for mild and asymptomatic hypertension as well. Investigators hope that the Australian therapeutic trial of mild hypertension and the current British Medical Research Council trial of the treatment of mild hypertension will establish the blood-pressure at which treatment is worthwhile (*Lancet* 1980). With the prospect of many more people in the community being identified as hypertensive than ever before, it is important to bear in mind that the labelling of someone as hypertensive and the use of anti-hypertensive drugs can have adverse effects which themselves may be disabling.

In Lambeth, hypertension was associated with restrictions in eating and drinking and in recreation and pastime. For example, hypertensive people are often advised to avoid salt, rest more, and not take part in strenuous pastimes. Some evidence suggests that labelling someone as hypertensive can cause psychiatric symptoms. Bloom and Monterossa (1981) found that normotensive people who were not receiving hypotensive therapy, but had been told in a screening survey that they were hypertensive, were more depressed and felt less well than the other normotensive people. Mann (1977) reported that people who had been told that they were hypertensive seemed to show more hostility than controls, whereas there was no relation between blood-pressure and psychiatric illness among people simply being screened for hypertension. There is little information about the amount of disability that can be caused by the depression and hostility resulting from labelling someone as hypertensive. Haynes *et al.* (1978) showed that the detection and labelling of hypertensive employees in an industrial setting without counselling can result in increased absenteeism.

The results from the Lambeth survey suggest that depression is another area in which hypertension is associated with disability. There is evidence that labelling someone as hypertensive does not result in depression if it is followed by reassurance and treatment. Bulpitt *et al.* (1976) found no difference in the amount of depression between patients receiving treatment in a hospital clinic for hypertension and controls. Yet, people newly referred to the hospital for hypertension who were studied before the start of treatment were more depressed than the controls.

Depression was associated with disability in many areas of life. As mentioned above, depression may be the cause of disability or the result of it. Evidence is scarce for the effectiveness of the primary prevention of depression. Certain measures can be taken, however, since there is growing evidence for a causative or at least precipitating relationship between stress and the development of psychiatric symptoms (Brown and Birley 1968; Brown *et al.* 1977; Brown *et al.* 1973). Possible measures include counselling services for the middle-aged, retired, and elderly; support for people with chronic or acute incapacitating diseases and disorders, and mutilating injuries; suicide prevention; and centres provided by voluntary groups such as the Samaritans who are available 24 hours a day for people in distress (Department of Health and Social Security 1976). However, the effectiveness of these measures in reducing depression has not been properly evaluated in randomized controlled trials.

The Lambeth Health Survey showed that only a few symptoms that were unreported or untreated were associated with disability and only for one or two activities. Moreover, respondents with unreported or untreated disabling symptoms were generally less restricted than respondents who had reported the same symptoms to their doctors and/or who were receiving treatment for them. Thus, there appears to be little possibility of preventing disability in Lambeth by increasing doctors' awareness and treatment of disabling symptoms. Nevertheless, the level of disability in the population may be reduced by improving the quality of care that disabled respondents receive from their general practitioners. Information about the sort of treatment that disabled respondents in Lambeth received after consulting their general practitioner is presented in Chapter 6.

Note

A full discussion of the relationship between impairment and disability can be found in: Peach, H. *The relationship between impairment and disability in disabled persons in the community*. PhD. Thesis, University of London.

References

Alderman, M. H. and Davies, T. K. (1976). Hypertensive control at the work site. *Journal of Occupational Medicine* **18**, 793–6.

Bennett, A. E. and Garrad, J. (1970). Chronic disease and disability in the community: a prevalence study. *British Medical Journal* **3**, 762–4.

Bloom, J. R. and Monterossa, S. (1981). Hypertension labelling and sense of well-being. *American Journal of Public Health* **71**, 1228–32.

Brown, G. W. and Birley, J. L. T. (1968). Crises and life changes and the onset of schizophrenia. *Journal of Health and Social Behaviour* **9**, 203–14.

Brown, G. W., Harris, T. O., and Copeland, J. R. (1977). Depression and loss. *British Journal of Psychiatry* **130**, 1–18.

Brown, G. W., Harris, T. O., and Peto, J. (1973). Life events and psychiatric disorder: nature of causal link. *Psychological Medicine* **3**, 150–76.

Bulpitt, C. J., Dollery, C. T., and Carne, S. (1976). Change in symptoms of hypertensive patients after referral to hospital clinics. *British Heart Journal* **38**, 121–8.

Chen, M. K. and Buck, R. D. (1981). Measuring the health care needs of an adult population in California. *Medical Care* **19**, 452–64.

DeJong, G. and Lifchez R. (1983). Physical disability and public policy. *Scientific American* **246**, 40–9.

Department of Health and Social Security (1976). *Prevention: everybody's business.* HMSO, London.

Dunnell, K. and Cartwright, A. (1972). *Medicine takers, prescribers and hoaders.* Routledge and Kegan Paul, London.

Harris, A. I. (1971). *Handicapped and impaired in Great Britain.* HMSO, London.

Haynes, R. B., Sackett, D. L., Taylor, W., Gibson, E. S., and Johnson, A. L. (1978). Increased absenteeism from work after detection and labelling of hypertensive patients. *New England Journal of Medicine* **299**, 741–4.

Ingham, J. G. and Miller, P.McC. (1979). Symptom prevalence and severity in a general practice population. *Journal of Epidemiology and Community Health* **33**, 191–8.

Lancet (1980). The pressure to treat. *Lancet* **1**, 1283–4.

Mann, A. H. (1977). The psychological effect of a screening programme and clinical trial for hypertension upon the participants. *Psychological Medicine* **7**, 431–8.

Morrell, D. C. and Wale, C. J. (1976). Symptoms perceived and recorded by patients. *Journal of the Royal College of General Practitioners* **27**, 398–403.

Stocks, P. (1949). *Sickness in the population of England and Wales in 1944–7.* General register office studies on medical and population subjects No. 2. HMSO, London.

Wadsworth, M. E. J., Butterfield W. J., and Blaney, R. (1971). *Health and sickness: the choice of treatment.* Tavistock, London.

Warren, M. (1974). *The Canterbury study of handicapped people*. Health Services Research Unit, University of Kent, Canterbury.

Williamson, J., Stoke, I. H., Gray, S., Fisher, M., Smith, A., McGhee, A., and Stephenson, E. (1964). Old people at home: their unreported needs. *Lancet* **1**, 1117–20.

6

Disability and iatrogenesis

HEDLEY PEACH

In the most narrow sense, iatrogenic disease includes only illnesses that would not have come about if sound and professionally recommended treatment had not been applied. In a more general and more widely accepted sense, clinical iatrogenic disease comprises all clinical conditions for which remedies, physicians, or hospitals are the pathogens, or 'sickening' agents. Medicines have always been potentially poisonous, but their unwanted side-effects have increased with their power and widespread use. Every 24 to 36 hours, from 50 to 80 per cent of adults in the United States and the United Kingdom swallow a medically-prescribed chemical.

Ivan Illich, *Medical Nemesis*, 1976

Disabled people who participated in the Lambeth Health Survey were heavy users of both general practitioner and hospital services. Thirty one per cent of disabled respondents had consulted their general practitioner within 3 weeks preceding the first interview. Fifty per cent of the disabled had attended casualty or out-patients within 9 months of the first interview, and 22 per cent had been a hospital in patient in the last year. Table 6.1 shows that out of 251 patient-initiated consultations with general practitioners, 134 (53 per cent) were to get a prescription. The prescribing of drugs was the most frequent service which general practitioners gave to disabled patients with 200 of the consultations resulting in a prescription. In addition, 15 per cent of the respondents visited their doctor's surgery to pick up a prescription for themselves without talking to the doctor.

Disabled respondents were asked whether they were satisfied with different aspects of care provided by general practitioners. Being disabled did not appear to be associated with negative evaluations of doctors (Patrick *et al.* 1983); in fact, disabled respondents were less likely to be dissatisfied with doctors than

Table 6.1. *General practitioner services sought by and provided for disabled people*

Service	Number of consultations	
	Sought	Provided
Prescribing of drugs	134	200
Physical examination	31	68
Advice or reassurance	18	42
Certificate	14	24
Injection or immunization	8	10
Referral to hospital	0	22
Ordering of appliance or aids	0	2

$N = 251$ consultations

those without any disability, perhaps arising from their long experience with medical care providers. However, respondents with and without disability expressed dissatisfaction with health education and information about disease and illness provided by doctors suggesting that patients expect the medical profession to play a greater part in health promotion.

The majority of patients also expressed satisfaction when asked about their own doctor. However, what dissatisfaction there was tended to be greater among respondents with disability than those without disability. Patients with disability are likely to be more dependent on their specific doctor for improvement or maintenance of their health. Again the main area of dissatisfaction for respondents with and without disability was the amount of information their own doctor had given them about their health.

Disabled people in the Lambeth Health Survey appeared to be satisfied with a mode of care comprised mainly of the prescribing of drugs. However, and perhaps unknown to many disabled people, reliance on drugs can also lead to problems of its own. Our data indicate that iatrogenic symptoms are common among disabled persons in Lambeth. For a large proportion of respondents, care was being provided by both hospital clinicians and the general practitioner. This division of care often means that neither the hospital consultant nor the general practitioner has primary responsibility for prescribing. Second, disabled respondents were taking nine times as many drugs as the non-disabled; most (87 per cent) of the drugs had been prescribed by a doctor (Peach 1984). There were only a small number of symptoms which respondents were treating themselves. In fact, there were only four respondent-treated symptoms where the frequency was greater than 3 per cent in any age group of either men or women. These were headaches; toothache, pain in jaw or sore gums; dry cough or sore throat; and constipation.

The frequency with which prescribed drugs were being taken by disabled people in Lambeth was greater than had previously been found in a survey of all adults living at home. Dunnell and Cartwright (1972), in their survey of a random sample of adult electors in 14 constituencies in England, Wales and Scotland, found that only two-thirds of consultations over a 2-week period resulted in a prescription. Only 41 per cent of the adults in their survey were taking a prescribed drug although 67 per cent were taking a non-prescribed drug.

Adverse drug reactions

An adverse reaction to a drug has been defined as 'any unintended or undesired consequence of drug therapy' (Cluff *et al.* 1964) or, alternatively, as any effect of a drug that is 'noxious and unintended and occurs at doses in man for prophylaxis, investigation, or therapy' (World Health Organization 1969). Reactions have been classified in terms of the probability of their causation by a drug into 'documented', 'probable' and 'possible' adverse reactions (Seidl *et al.* 1965). A 'documented' adverse reaction is one commonly known to occur with a definite temporal relationship to taking the drug and a positive re-challenge test or laboratory confirmation. A probable reaction is one commonly known to occur with a definite temporal association and improvement on withdrawal of the drug. A possible reaction is one that is known to occur, but the temporal relationship is less clear, and other causes are possible.

Prevalance of adverse drug reactions

Several surveys have dealt with the incidence of adverse drug reactions in hospital practice. Hurwitz (1969) and Hurwitz and

Wade (1969) observed 1268 in-patients in two Belfast hospitals, and drug reactions were found in 10 per cent of all patients receiving drug therapy (digitalis, ampicillin, and bronchodilators, particularly). In medical wards the incidence was 16 per cent. Of the 129 reactions to drugs reported by Hurwitz and Wade (1969), 6 reactions were classified as 'documented', 118 as 'probable', and 5 as 'possible'. Hurwitz and Wade compared their results with those of other hospital surveys in Canada and the USA, and found incidence rates of between 1 per cent and 18 per cent. Most of the surveys reviewed by Hurwitz and Wade and those published since then, also mainly Canadian or American, have found incidence rates of between 10 and 20 per cent (Slone *et al.* 1966, Jick *et al.* 1970, Borda *et al.* 1968). The variation in incidence rate is due, in part, to the different age and sex structure of the hospital populations studied, the survey designs (some have been prospective and others retrospective) and the method of recording adverse drug reactions.

There have been fewer surveys of adverse drug reactions in the community. The hospital survey conducted by Hurwitz and Wade found that 3 per cent of the 1268 patients seen were admitted to the hospital because of an adverse reaction to a drug taken at home for therapeutic reasons. Among the drugs which caused such adverse reactions were digitalis preparations, antibiotics, corticosteroids, anticoagulants, analgestics, and tranquillizers. In a year's survey of adverse drug reactions in a general practice, Mulroy (1973) found that 1 consultation in every 40 was the result of an adverse reaction to a drug. Both 'probable' and 'possible' adverse drug reactions were included. The proportion of consultations due to adverse drug reactions was greater among women than men and as great among 40–59-year-olds as among the elderly. Clearly, adverse drug reactions among patients not consulting would not have been included. Martys (1979) used a doctor-administered questionnaire to elicit adverse drug reactions over 12 months among patients in a general practice who received an antibiotic, a drug acting on the central nervous, cardiorespiratory, or gastrointestinal systems, an antihistamine, and a nutritional, hormonal, or metabolic drug for the first time and who were not taking any other drug. Of the 817 patients who received a drug in one of these groups the incidence of 'documented' and 'probable' adverse reactions was 41 per cent.

The most widely used classification of the severity of adverse drug reactions (Seidl *et al.* 1965) does not distinguish between the impact of the drug reaction on the life of the patient and the consequences for future drug therapy. A 'severe' drug reaction is considered to be one which is fatal or life-threatening; a 'moderate' drug reaction is considered to be one which requires treatment, admission to hospital, or prolongs the stay in hospital by at least a day; and a 'mild' drug reaction is considered to be one which is incidental, requires no treatment, and does not necessarily call for withdrawal of treatment. In the survey conducted by Hurwitz and Wade 80 per cent of the adverse drug reactions were considered to be moderate. No information exists on the severity of adverse drug reactions in the community, nor on the amount of disability caused by adverse drug reactions either in hospital or in the community.

Possible adverse drug reactions in Lambeth

The drugs being taken most frequently by disabled adults in Lambeth were analgesics, diuretics, sedatives, hypnotics, and tranquillizers. Some of the symptoms that were found to account for most of the disability in Lambeth (Chapter 5) are known to be adverse effects of the drugs being taken most frequently by disabled persons (Table 6.2). Some commonly prescribed analgesics, for example, aspirin, codeine, or dihydrocodeine, are known to cause stomach pain, constipation, or giddiness (Joint Formularly Committee 1981*a*). Diuretics can disturb sleep and promote or aggravate incontinence. Some commonly prescribed diuretics, for example, frusemide can cause general tiredness or weakness (Bailey 1980). Antidepressants can cause spells of giddiness (Joint Formulary Committee 1981*b*). Sedatives have been said to cause trouble learning, remembering, or thinking clearly; difficulty keeping balance on feet; and general tiredness or weakness (Joint Formulary Committee 1981*c*).

A significantly higher proportion of respondents who complained of spells of giddiness, stomach pain, and constipation were taking analgesics than those respondents without those symptoms. Similarly, a significantly higher proportion of respondents who had difficulty keeping their balance; general tiredness or weakness; and trouble learning, remembering, or thinking clearly, were

Table 6.2. *Possible relationship between disabling symptoms and drugs being taken by disabled people in Lambeth*

Disabling symptom	Drugs which could cause symptom
Difficulty getting to sleep or staying asleep at night	Diuretics
Difficulty keeping balance on feet	Sedatives
General tiredness or weakness	Diuretics
Trouble learning, remembering, or thinking clearly	Sedatives
Limbs paralysed, deformed, missing, or broken	
Pain or stiffness in joints or back	
Swelling of feet or ankles	
Shortness of breath	
Trouble seeing, hearing, or talking	
Constipation	Analgesics
Loss of appetite or weight	
Pain in stomach	Analgesics
Pain in calves	
Frequency or incontinence of urine	Diuretics
Spells of feeling hot, nervous, or shaky	
Spells of giddiness	Analgesics, antidepressants

taking sedatives. Furthermore, a significantly higher proportion of respondents complaining of spells of giddiness and trouble learning, remembering, or thinking clearly were taking antidepressants than respondents not complaining of such symptoms.

Possible adverse drug reactions and disability in Lambeth

Repondents who complained of difficulty getting to sleep or staying asleep at night and frequency or incontinence of urine, and who were taking diuretics, were significantly more disabled than respondents with those symptoms not taking diuretics (Table 6.3). Similarly respondents complaining of difficulty keeping their balance; trouble learning, remembering, or thinking clearly; and general tiredness or weakness, and who were taking sedatives,

Table 6.3. *Relationship between symptoms, drugs, and category scores of the Functional Limitations Profile*

Symptom and drug	Communication	Eating and drinking	Body care and movement of limbs	Ambulation	Mobility	Household management	Rest	Recreation and pastime	Social interaction
Difficulty getting to sleep or staying asleep at night + diuretics			0.05	0.67	0.57	1.06	1.78	0.99	0.64
Difficulty keeping balance on feet + sedatives			0.08	2.40	1.66	2.18	1.48	2.39	1.07
General tiredness or weakness + sedatives					2.83	0.67	1.27	1.09	1.04
Trouble learning, remembering, or thinking clearly + sedatives	1.67					1.07	2.75	1.35	1.11
Constipation + analgesics		0.53						0.80	
Pain in stomach between meals or disturbing sleep + analgesics								1.63	
Frequency or incontinence of urine + diuretics			0.08	0.59	1.23		1.53	0.87	0.69

were more disabled than respondents with those symptoms who were not taking sedatives. Respondents with stomach pain or constipation taking analgesics were more disabled than respondents with stomach pain or constipation not taking analgesics. Respondents with unreported or untreated giddiness and taking analgesics or antidepressants were more disabled than respondents with giddiness who were not taking either analgesics or antidepressants.

As defined previously a possible adverse drug reaction is one that is known to occur, but the temporal relationship is unclear and other causes are possible. Diuretics are known to contribute to frequency or incontinence of urine and analgesics are known to cause or aggravate constipation and stomach pain. However, information about when the respondents started to take diuretics and analgesics and when they developed frequency or incontinence of urine, constipation, and stomach pain was not collected during the Lambeth survey. It is also difficult to exclude other possible causes for relationships between diuretics and analgesics and frequency or incontinence of urine, constipation, and stomach pain, when the information about symptoms and drugs have been collected by lay interviews in a health survey. Lay interviewers cannot probe to exclude other causes of these symptoms. Therefore, it is difficult to do more than identify restrictions in life which might possibly be the adverse effect of diuretics and analgesics. By further analysis of the data it was possible to test other explanations for the association between taking diuretics and the reporting of difficulty sleeping, and between taking sedatives and the reporting of difficulty keeping balance on feet; trouble learning, remembering, or thinking clearly; and tiredness.

It has been assumed that difficulty sleeping is an adverse effect of diuretics which cause the patient to get up at night to pass urine. However, the association between difficulty sleeping and diuretics would also occur if the cause was breathlessness when lying flat in bed because of the heart disease for which the patient was taking diuretics.

There are two pieces of evidence against the latter interpretation. First, interactions between difficulty sleeping and diuretics were positively associated with all categories of disability except for eating and communication. However, Chatper 5 showed that heart trouble was associated with only one category and that was eating. Bronchitis and therefore possibly cor pulmonale, was associated only with ambulation. Asthma, often indistinguishable from bronchitis, was associated with only recreation and pastime. If shortness of breath consequent upon heart disease was responsible for the difficulty in sleeping, then the congression of disability on diseases or disorders would have shown that heart disease or bronchitis was associated with more than just two categories of disability. Second, if the association between diuretics and difficulty sleeping was spurious, as described above, one would expect the taking of diuretics among respondents with difficulty sleeping and shortness of breath to be greater than among those complaining of only difficulty sleeping. In fact the proportion of respondents taking diuretics was the same in both groups.

The association between taking sedatives and problems of balance, thinking, and tiredness could have come about because the psychological problem for which the doctor prescribed sedatives included these symptoms and not because the symptoms were caused by the sedatives being taken. If the sedative were causing problems of balance, thinking, and tiredness, then the taking of sedatives should have been greater among depressed or anxious respondents complaining of those symptoms than among depressed or anxious patients without those symptoms. In fact, the taking of sedatives was no greater among depressed or anxious patients without problems of balance, thinking, and tiredness than among respondents with those symptoms. It seems likely, there-fore, that the sedatives were causing the problems of balance, thinking, and tiredness.

There is a lot of literature available on the trends in psycho-tropic drug prescribing and addiction to and self-poisoning by this group of drugs. Therefore, the suggestion that any association between disability and sedatives is unlikely to be spurious might seem surprising. In fact there have been few studies of the amount of disability caused by sedatives and tranquillizers with which to compare the results of the Lambeth study. Skegg *et al.* (1979) showed that patients taking minor tranquillizers have an increased risk of road accidents, but failed to distinguish between the effects of the drug and the psychological condition for which the drugs were prescribed. Eelkema *et al.* (1970) suggested that patients were less likely to be injured on the roads after treatment in a mental hospital than before treatment. Most of the evidence that sedatives and tranquillizers impair motor skills comes from studies of volunteers in laboratory situations. Landauer (1981) has recently reviewed these studies and concludes that none of them give a clear indication as to whether orally-administered diazepam adversely affects the ability to drive a car. Overstall *et al.* (1977) found no association between the prescribing of sedatives and difficulty in keeping balance among the elderly.

In Lambeth, difficulty getting to sleep or staying asleep at night and frequency or incontinence of urine were associated with restriction in many areas of life. It was possible that these symptoms were the adverse effects of diuretics and many of the hypertensive respondents were taking diuretics. Bulpitt and Dollery (1973), using a self-administered symptom questionnaire, found that between 33 and 57 per cent of patients being treated at a hypertensive clinic with diuretics alone and in combination with other drugs complained of 'sleeplessness'. Jachurst *et al.* (1982) assess the quality of life after antihypertensive therapy in 75 patients with controlled hypertension using questionnaires given to patients, close companions, and doctors. The questionnaire completed by relatives rated 19 (25 per cent) of patients to have suffered mild adverse changes, 33 (45 per cent) to have had moderate adverse changes and 22 patients (30 per cent) severe adverse changes.

The data from the Lambeth survey, like that of Bulpitt and Dollery (1973) and Jachurst *et al.* (1982), can only point to possible adverse effects of drugs. Any investigation of the incidence of iatrogenic symptoms and disability is affected by the 'non-drug' reaction. Reidenberg and Lowenthal (1968) have shown that a positive history of many symptoms commonly considered to be drug side-effects can be elicited from healthy people who are not taking any medication. This emphasizes the importance of the doctor being aware of all pre-existing symptoms and physical signs before starting treatment so that the symptoms and signs the patient's attention are drawn to after treatment has started may not be erroneously labelled as side-effects.

As epidemiologists we must necessarily be cautious when interpreting statistically significant associations between the reporting of symptoms and the taking of specific drugs because such correlations could be spurious. However, there was good circumstantial evidence for iatrogenic symptoms being common in

Lambeth. This evidence, together with statistically significant associations between the taking of analgesics and giddiness or constipation and between the taking of diuretics and difficulty sleeping, are compelling grounds for further research to be undertaken in this area.

A final word of caution is necessary. Disability and iatrogenesis is a very difficult area. Even if it could be proved conclusively that some of the disabling symptoms reported in Lambeth were adverse reactions to the drugs being taken, it would not follow that the level of disability would necessarily be reduced by withdrawing the offending drug from the patients' treatment regimes. A reduction in disability would only occur if the disabling effect of the untreated symptom was less than that of the adverse drug reaction. However, general practitioners might be able to substitute an equally effective drug, which does not cause an adverse reaction, for the drug which has disabling side-effects. This pre-supposes that the general practitioners are aware of the drugs being taken by their disabled patients. Information about medication being taken by a random sample of disabled patients of all ages in a group practice was compared with the entries in their general practitioners' records and doctors' working knowledge (from memory and records) of the drugs that their patients were taking (Patrick *et al.* 1982, Peach 1983). The doctors knew of only 64 per cent of the drugs the patients told the interviewers they were taking. It would be worth general practitioners' while considering ways of improving their knowledge of what medication their patients are taking, particularly as some of the symptoms among their disabled patients might be adverse drug reactions.

Note

A full discussion of the relationship between adverse drug reactions and disability can be found in Peach H. *The relationship between impairment and disability among disabled persons in the community.* PhD Thesis University of London, 1984.

References

Bailey, W. A. J. M. (1980). *Data sheet compendium 1980–1* Data Pharm Publications Limited, London. Page 419.

Borda, I. T., Slone, D., and Jick, H. (1968). Assessment of adverse reactions within a drug surveillance programme. *Journal of the American Medical Association* **205**, 645–7.

Bulpitt, C. J. and Dollery, C. T. (1973). Side-effects of hypotensive agents evaluated by a self-administered questionnaire. *British Medical Journal* **3**, 485–90.

Cluff, L. E., Thornton, G. F., and Seidl, L. G. (1964). Studies on the epidemiology of adverse drug reactions: methods of survillance. *Journal of the American Medical Association* **188**, 976–83.

Dunnell, K. and Cartwright, A. (1972). *Medicine takers, prescribers and hoarders*. Routledge and Kegan Paul, London.

Eelkema, R. C., Brosseaus, J., Koshnick, R., and McGee, C. (1970). A statistical study on the relationship between mental illness and traffic accidents—a pilot study. *American Journal of Public Health* **60**, 459–63.

Hurwitz, N. (1969). Admission to hospital due to drugs. *British Medical Journal* **1**, 539–40.

Hurwitz, N. and Wade, O. L. (1969). Intensive hospital monitoring of adverse reactions to drugs. *British Medical Journal* **1**, 521–6.

Jachurst, S. J., Brierley, H., Jachurst, S., and Wilcox, P. M. (1982). The effect of hypertensive drugs on the quality of life. *Journal of Royal College of General Practitioners* **32**, 103–5.

Jick, H., Meittinen, O. S., Shapiro, S., Lewis, G. P., Siskind, V., and Slone, D. (1970). Comprehensive drug surveillance. *The Journal of American Medical Association* **213**, 1455–60.

Joint Formulary Committee (1981*a*). *British National Formularly*. British Medical Association and the Pharmaceutical Society of Great Britain, London. Pages 128–33.

Joint Formularly Committee (1981*b*). *British National Formularly*. British Medical Association and the Pharmaceutical Society of Great Britain, London. Pages 115–22.

Joint Formularly Committee (1981*c*). *British National Formularly*. British Medical Association and the Pharmaceutical Society of Great Britain, London. Pages 100–7.

Landauer, A. A. (1981). Diazepam and driving ability. *Medical Journal of Australia* **1**, 624–6.

Martys, C. R. (1979). Adverse reactions to drugs in general practice. *British Medical Journal* **2**, 1194–7.

Mulroy, R. (1973). Iatrogenic disease in general practice: its incidence and effects. *British Medical Journal* **2**, 407–10.

Overstall, P. W., Exton-Smith, A. N., Imms, G. J., and Johnson, A. L. (1977). Falls in the elderly related to postural imbalance. *British Medical Journal* **1**, 261–4.

Patrick, D. L., Peach, H., and Gregg, I. (1982). Disablement and care: a comparison of patient views and general practitioner knowledge. *Journal of the Royal College of General Practitioners* **32**, 429–34.

Patrick, D. L., Scrivens, E., and Charlton, J. (1983). Disability and patient satisfaction with medical care. *Medical Care* **21**, 1062–75.

Peach, H. (1983). Trends in self-prescribing and attitudes to self-medication. *Practitioner* **227**, 1609–15.

Peach, H. (1984). The relative contribution of physician and self-medication in the drug treatment of symptoms. In *Symposium on self-medication* (ed. L. E. Fryklof and R. Westerling). Swedish Pharmaceutical Press, Stockholm.

Reidenberg, M. M. and Lowenthal, D. T. (1968). Adverse non-drug reactions. *New England Journal of Medicine* **279**, 678–9.

Seidl, L. G., Thornton, G. F., and Cluff, L. E. (1965). Epidemiological studies of adverse drug reactions. *American Journal of Public Health* **55**, 1170–5.

Skegg, D. C. G., Richards, S. M., and Doll, R. (1979). Minor tranqillisers and road accidents. *British Medical Journal* **1**, 917–9.

Slone, D., Jick, H., Borda, I., *et al.* (1966). Drug surveillance utilising nurse monitors. *Lancet* **2**, 901–3.

World Health Organization (1969). Technical Services Report Number 425. World Health Organization, Geneva.

7

Allocating resources to meet needs

DONALD L. PATRICK AND ELLIE SCRIVENS

> In a society in which there is genuine respect for the
> handicapped; where understanding is unostentatious and
> sincere; where if years cannot be added to the lives of the very
> sick, at least life can be added to their years; where needs
> come before means; where the mobility of disabled people is
> restricted only by the bounds of technical progress and
> discovery; where the handicapped have a fundamental right
> to participate in industry and society according to ability;
> where socially preventable distress is unknown; and where no
> man has cause to feel ill-at-ease because of his disability.
>
> Alf Morris in presenting the bill for the chronically Sick and
> Disabled Persons Act for the second reading

In Chapter 1 we discussed the use of survey data to assess the need
for community resources among disabled persons, in terms of felt,
expressed, normative, and comparative needs. Most self-reported
information from interview surveys can be used to define
categories of felt or expressed needs, that is the desires and
demands for services or benefits. Survey information on the
current provision for disabled people or their status can be used to
assess comparative need as it relates to the broader community.
For example, if the income, education, mobility, or employment
levels of disabled people are lower than those of the general
population in a community, then disabled people can be considered
to have comparative needs. The allocation of resources to meet
felt, expressed, or comparative needs, is not a straightforward
task, however. Whether resources can be directed to meet
particular needs is a matter of policy and priorities. Whether the
provision is to be in cash or in kind also is an important issue. This

chapter describes how survey information can provide an assessment of resource need. We will use allocation of aids to daily living as a specific example of needs assessment. In addition, present State provisions in cash and in kind for disabled people in Britain will be examined in light of public opinion and the current resource allocation and rationing process.

Assessing need for daily living aids

For the last three decades, the British public has been able to receive health and personal social services free of charge or at below cost. Access to these services is universal and, for the most part, voluntary. Any individual who wishes to use a service can apply to that service for help. Providers, using eligibility criteria, professional assessment, or both, determine how the service can best help this individual. Their main concern is to meet the needs of the individual by supplying services or cash. Because the need for provision is determined initially by the individual, managers of the service do not know whether all eligible persons are receiving help. Community surveys have been used to determine public perceptions of particular needs, of the benefit of provisions, and of satisfaction with current provision. One of the objectives of the Lambeth Health Survey was to examine the need for and use of aids to daily living by disabled people residing in the community. The Functional Limitations Profile (FLP), described in chapters 3 and 4, was used to develop a measure of baseline need, that is an assessment of disability level or health status against which provisions could be evaluated and measured. Each FLP statement describes a dysfunctional behaviour, for example: 'I make difficult movements with help, such as getting in and out of the bath', which can be compared with the availability, use, and need for aids. Respondents who reported that they experienced functional limitations were asked about their use of and need for all the aids available from the social services departments that have responsibility for Lambeth residents. Respondents were shown photographs of the aids while being asked the following questions:

1. Do you have any need for aids to help you with this behaviour (for example, to dress)?
2. If yes, do you use the aid?

3. Do you need any additional aids (to help you dress)?
4. If yes, have you applied to the local authority for them?

The responses to these questions showed the proportion of the respondents who had aids, used them, wanted them, and/or had applied for them. These responses were then used to classify respondents according to the different dimensions of need defined in Table 7.1. These dimensions expand the categories of need previously described to include unrecognized, satisfied, and acceptably and unacceptably met needs.

Table 7.1. *Categories of need for aids to daily living reported by disabled respondents in Lambeth*

Category of need	Definition: respondent reported
Felt	Functional limitation present, aids to help and aids used.
Expressed	Functional limitation present, perceived need for aids, and aids applied for.
Comparative	Functional limitation present, but no aids to help.
Unrecognized	Functional limitation present, no aids to help and no perceived need for aids.
Satisfied	Functional limitation present, aids to help and no perceived needs for additional aids.
Acceptably met need	Functional limitation present, aids to help and aids used.
Unacceptably met need	Functional limitation present, aids to help but Not used.

Fig. 7.1 illustrates the number of disabled people who perceived need for aids to help with 'trouble putting on shoes, socks, or stockings'. The aids for this particular limitation include shoe horns and stocking applicators. Almost 89 per cent of those who stated they experienced this limitation had no dressing aids to help them, meaning that their comparative need was high. Unrecognized need, defined as reporting a limitation but not feeling that aids could help, also was high (83.2 per cent), indicating that few people without dressing aids felt they could benefit from them.

Comparing satisfied need with appropriately met need indicates that those who used aids to help with dressing did not feel they needed more. However, the proportion of respondents who reported that they wanted aids but had not applied to the local authority for them was greater than the proportion of those who had applied.

Fig. 7.2 shows the categories of perceived need associated with 'moving hands or fingers with some difficulty or limitation'. The aids for this limitation include special can openers, tap-turners, or

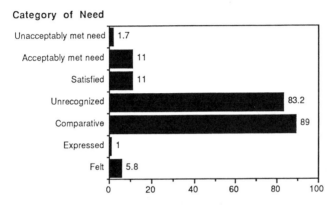

Fig. 7.1 Proportion of respondents reporting need for aids to assist putting on shoes, socks or stockings.

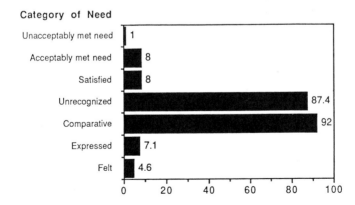

Fig. 7.2. Proportion of respondents reporting need for aids to assist with hand or finger movements.

levers, and special cooking aids. Again, comparative need was high (92 per cent), but less than 5 per cent perceived that they could benefit from such aids. Satisfied need and appropriately met needs were the same (8 per cent), indicating that those who used their aids did not feel they required additional help.

Fig. 7.3 shows the reported needs related to 'making difficult movements with help, for example, getting in and out of the bath'. The aids for this limitation include a bath step, bath hoist, and bath board. The proportion of the sample classified as having comparative need here was lower than for the previous two examples (under 80 per cent), mainly because unrecognized need was lower (76 per cent) such that few respondents perceived any benefit from having these aids. The majority of disabled people who had bathing aids used them (21.5 per cent), compared with those who did not (2 per cent).

Category of Need

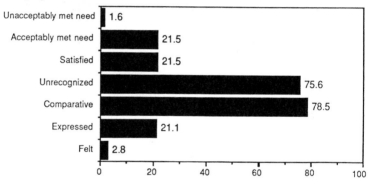

Fig. 7.3. Proportion of respondents reporting need for aids to assist with getting into or out of the bath.

Table 7.2 summarizes the reported needs for aids to daily living associated with four other specific functional limitations. For most daily living aids, the pattern of needs within the community was similar. The existence of comparative need was explained most often by the extent of unrecognized need. In addition, very few people who had aids wanted more of them.

Many people who reported limitations in function or activity restrictions did not perceive a need for aids. High levels of

Table 7.2. *Proportion of respondents with needs for aids to daily living by specific functional limitation*

Needs	Felt %	Expressed %	Comparative %	Unrecognized %	Satisfied %	Acceptable %	Unacceptable %	Total N
Moving in bed lifting/ monkey pole/hoists/rope/ ladder	3.9	1	98.7	94.8	1.3	1.3	0	77
Difficulty moving in/out of bed monkey pole/rope ladder	3.3	1	99.6	96.3	1	3.3	0	248
Walking and using stairs/ sticks/walking frames	0	3.9	61.5	61.5	37.9	38.5	8.3	314
Kneel, stoop, or bend by holding aids for getting in/out of bath	14.7	1.8	81.1	66.4	19.1	5.1	1.5	333

unrecognized need suggest further investigation about the knowledge of eligibility for services and access to services. Comparing satisfied needs with inappropriately met needs indicates the proportion of people who are not satisfied with the amount of service they receive in relation to those who are satisfied. Most Lambeth respondents were satisfied with the provision of daily living aids. Comparing inappropriately met need with appropriately met need makes it possible to identify the proportion of people who have aids that they do not use. Social service providers are very concerned with unused aids. It has been suggested that if unused aids were reclaimed by the issuing authority, they could be allocated to others who would use them. The Lambeth data suggest, however, that the number of people possessing aids but not using them is low. Thus, it is doubtful whether an effort to locate unused aids would be justified.

This taxonomy of needs can be used to provide information for many disablement services, using survey questions specially constructed for the different services to which they applied. In the case of home-help service, for example, a baseline of need could be established by asking questions about respondents' ability to shop and do housework. Unrecognized need could then be established by enquiring about the perceived need for home help, and other needs could be assessed following the format described for aids to daily living.

Service managers must decide what levels of service provision they wish to achieve and to what extent consumers should and could influence their allocations. Comparing different dimensions of need for different provisions and services can help providers determine what actions to take. Service providers who know their own methods of provision and the characteristics of the communities in which they work must determine why different types of need exist.

Service provision can often be a rigid process that meets specific and limited needs. A different pattern of provision or new provisions might be more beneficial to disabled people and to their families. All respondents in Phase I of the Lambeth Health Survey were asked if they would like to make suggestions for helping disabled people. Overall, 535 respondents (402 disabled and 133 non-disabled) made nearly 700 suggestions. The most frequently offered suggestion was for financial assistance of one kind or another (7.4 per cent of all suggestions). Other frequently offered suggestions included someone to call regularly (5.8 per cent), more ramps in streets and buildings (5.2 per cent), and additional housing and maintenance services (4.5 per cent). Eight per cent of disabled respondents and 3 per cent of non-disabled respondents offering suggestions felt that disabled persons had sufficient services and benefits at that time.

Information on service needs obtained from community surveys is admittedly crude, but it is useful in that it uncovers problems that exist in allocating provisions. Investigating reasons for different perceptions of needs in a community can lead to specific actions or changes in the system of provision. The information derived from survey data also can be presented in a simple and interesting manner that is helpful in determining how well services cover the population in need and the acceptability or perceived usefulness of these services to the public.

Present State provisions for disabled people in Britain

There is no one policy that encompasses the provision of services or benefits for disabled people in Britain. Each provision caters to specifc aspects of life and is derived from a set of policy principles created by historical rather than logical determinants. The income maintenance system, for example, evolved separately from the many other provisions available to disabled people. Consequently, there are two independent systems for transfers of resources from the government to recipients: cash and services. These two systems reflect a number of different and often conflicting principles for resources allocation that have resulted in a bewilderingly complex system of community provision.

Cash benefits

The present system of cash benefits is founded on three basic principles that underlie the main legislative development upon which people with disabilities depend (Simpkins 1978). The first one is the insurance principle. It is the central feature of the British social security system in which payments are made from a person's earned income to provide for benefits in the event of unemployment or sickness. Employees, employers, and the State contribute to the funds. The majority of disabled people have contributed to the national scheme of insurance before acquiring a disability benefit, although those severely impaired or disabled from birth may not have paid into the system.

The second principle is that of the relief of destitution, the major element underlying the Poor Law Acts enacted under Queen Elizabeth I and in 1834. While public responsibility for relieving poverty was the goal of Poor Law legislation, the effect was to distinguish between the 'deserving' and 'undeserving' poor, since administration of the law required one to prove the most abject poverty before receiving assistance. Unemployment of an able-bodied person was regarded as the individual's own responsibility. Under the Poor Law some people perferred to starve rather than be part of the system's charity. While the system was not concerned directly with disabled people, the effect on those whose impairments prevented them from working was to make them a part of a stigmatized group along with able-bodied paupers.

The third principle, that of compensation, also developed with the growth of social security provision. The undesirable assistance from the Poor Law was a cause of grievance for those who experienced permanently incapacitating injuries at work, particularly when the injury stemmed from employer negligence. Compensation in the industrial context began as payment for loss of earnings due to employer negligence. The Workmen's Compensation Act of 1897 required employers in dangerous industries, such as coal mining, to provide income for permanently injured workmen if the employer was proved negligent in assuming worker safety. The onus of financial self-sufficiency and provision for the future thus was taken away from the individual and placed on the employer.

The principle of compensation for lost earnings was reinforced in war pensions, which go back as far as the sixteenth century, but which became more significant when large numbers of people became disabled during the 1914–18 war. War pensions were dependent upon the degree of injury or loss of functional ability and on rank. They were paid on top of earnings, introducing another important concept, that of compensation for disability over and above regular sources of income. In compensatory legislation after the First World War, the element of compensation for loss of earnings was combined with that of loss of faculty. Loss of faculty was the major determining factor of entitlement, calculated on a percentage of disability rising to 100 per cent. The loss of a foot, for example, was assessed as 30 per cent disablement. Disablement pensions, however, did not include any provision for additional expenses that resulted from disablement, either directly or indirectly.

A mixture of these principles of insurance, poverty relief, and compensation provided the basis for financial and social provisions in the years between the Workmen's Compensation Act and publication of the Beveridge Report in 1942. Compulsory health insurance for employees began in 1912, followed shortly by unemployment insurance in a few industries. The British Government and the unions in the 1920s and 1930s had heated debates about provisions for people injured at work. Industrial workers argued that they served their country as much as people who were injured at war, and thus were entitled to equivalent reward if an injury occurred at work. Separate provisions for specific types of disability also began, among the first of which was the Blind Persons Act of 1920. These welfare provisions were affected by changes in the medical system and in child care, as well as by the growth of trade union activity and friendly societies.

In 1942 Beveridge claimed that 'provision for most of the many varieties of need through interruption of earnings and other causes that may arise in modern industrial communities has already been made on a scale not surpassed and hardly rivalled in any other country'. The Beveridge Report was issued at a period when war was once again forcing many changes in social security provision. A 'reconstruction' period followed during which disabled people along with the entire community gained from major reforms such as government responsibility for maintaining full employment (1944), Family Allowances (1946), the National Health Service (1946), and the National Assistance Act (1948). These reforms implemented many of Beveridge's recommendations, including the fundamental principle of 'adequacy of benefit'. Shortcomings in the provisions were recognized in cases where the benefits were below the subsistence level, where they did not last as long as needed, or where they were supplemented by the administration of the dreaded means tests.

The National Assistance Act of 1948 was intended to provide for the limited number of cases where needs were not covered by social insurance. It contained an implicit respect for human dignity in that the legislation did not mandate any means test for an insurance benefit. The idea of introducing benefit at a level adequate for subsistence so that individuals could build upon a minimal guaranteed income was rejected, however. A total number of claimants and dependents eligible for national assistance or its equivalent rose from 1.5 million in 1948 to more than 4 million by 1970.

No logical long-term policy developed during the 1950s and 1960s to provide for disabled people. In 1966, earnings-related supplements were added to flat-rate sickness and industrial injury benefits, thus preventing an individual from suffering a decrease in standard of living through illness. Sickness benefits extend from the end of the second week of incapacity for a period of 26 weeks. This provision was intended to ease the transition from earnings to flat-rate benefits. If the illness still prevents a return to work, the individual claims invalidity pension, and if the illness begins before 60 years of age for men or 55 years for women, a supplement known as the invalidity allowance is added to the pension.

These invalidity allowances are small, but they introduced yet another principle into the income maintenance system—that of compensation for the age of onset of disability, without relation to the severity, type, or likely duration of disability. Until 1975 there was no payment as 'of right' in respect of disabilities except where those disabilities arose from war injuries, injury at work, or prescribed industrial disease. Further additions to the income maintenance provisions for disabled people have added still more principles by which individuals might be compensated. Mobility allowance was introduced to help those who, in the opinion of medical examiners, are not able to walk. This allowance has enabled disabled people to purchase help with mobility, such as paying for a car or taxi. The mobility allowance was introduce after considerable discussion over the value of special invalid cars to disabled people. Further patchwork provision was introduced with the attendance allowance, a benefit to help those who are severely disabled pay for substantial care by day or by night. Attendance allowance is paid as in case of attendance need, not in respect of disablement alone, thus becoming another specialized incapacity benefit. The more recent Non-Contributory Invalidity

Pension also is not paid in respect of disablement *per se*, but in respect to the inability to contribute to National Insurance.

In summary, a number of different principles have led to many direct lines of state provision involving monetary compensation to disabled people. These principles include:

1. The victim of sickness or disablement is provided with an income that will meet the essential requirements of a normally healthy person. As long as total incapacity for work is experienced, payments can be made through the supplementary benefits system to cover special needs that require increased expenditure, such as additional heating or clothing.
2. Individuals are compensated for loss of faculty due to either a specific incident or general medical conditions as in war and industrial injury pensions.
3. There are arbitrary tax concessions for the receipt of certain benefits, such as war pensions.
4. The law of damages provides arrangements for claims through the legal process.
5. Allowances for mobility and attendance are available along with the non-contributory pension schemes for people who cannot work and therefore cannot claim anything but supplementary benefit.

Services

As even broader mixture of philosophies and assumptions than those underlying monetary compensation have influenced the provision of services and goods to disabled people in Britain (Topliss 1982). Under the Poor Law, mentally and physically disabled people were provided for if they resided in the workhouse institutions, including access to food and medical care. At the end of the nineteenth century, social policy and service provisions concentrated on national efficiency by ensuring that all citizens could engage in productive employment. This emphasis on employment increased during the war when disabled people joined the industrial work force and when services were needed to take care of those injured in war.

Rehabilitation services were developed to meet the need for employing people disabled by war, including workshops explicitly for the disabled. At the end of the First World War, the policy thrust was almost entirely on retraining and employment. In 1920, service provisions were extended to one clearly impaired group: blind people. For all other groups of disabled people, material help was confined to provisions available under the Poor Law.

Similarly, in the Second World War, the major concern of social policy was on rehabilitation and training for employment. Disabled people who entered the severely depleted work force were taught new skills. In addition, a new category of disability was introduced, involving civilians who were injured in the war and needed certain services. The assumption that such services increased national efficiency was underscored by belief in the work ethic. The government also maintained that productive employment for disabled people would improve morale and possibly assist in curing them. From those perspectives came the now familiar services of occupational therapy and sheltered workshops. The Disabled Persons (Employment) Act of 1944, which remains in force, created a voluntary register of disabled persons wishing to work. The register is divided into those capable of working in open employment and those able to work only in sheltered workshops. This Act has provided assessment services, courses in rehabilitation centres, vocational retraining, and the help of a specialized professional known as the disablement resettlement officer. The Act also has required employers with 20 or more workers to employ a quota of 3 per cent registered disabled. These measures, designed to improve employment prospects of disabled people, have met with variable success through the rapidly shifting economic cycles of recent times (Manpower Services Commission 1981). (See Chapter 8 for a more complete discussion of work and disability.)

Other service provisions for disabled people were created by post-World War II legislation. The Poor Law was finally abandoned and replaced by a variety of Parliamentary Acts that covered a wide range of social provisions. In 1946 the National Heath Service Act made it possible for local authorities (who until 1984 were responsible for the provision of health services) to provide nursing care at home and to provide items such as aids to daily living that would help in the after-care of patients. The National Assistance Act of 1948 (Section 29) empowered local authorities to promote 'the welfare of persons . . . who are deaf or dumb and other persons who are substantially and permanently handicapped by illness, injury or congenital deformity, or such other disabilities as may be prescribed by the Minister'.

The tardiness of local authorities to implement schemes for providing the services specified by the National Assistance Act is well documented (Keeble 1979). It is not surprising that some authorities chose to rely on the provisions of voluntary organizations to meet their statutory requirements, since the legislation assumed that provisions could be made without any substantial increase in manpower. Skilled staff to evaluate the specific needs of disabled clients were few at the beginning of the 1950s, and few professional groups dealing with the special interests and needs of disabled people had evolved. The provisions of the legislation were by no means a 'right' of the people who needed them.

Throughout the two decades that followed the post-war legislation, local authorities 'muddled through'. The existence of particular services and their availability to any individual depended on the policy and finances of the relevant authority. In the critical area of housing, for example, disabled people fared better or worse depending on the housing stock, waiting lists, and administration practices of the various local authorities. During the 1950s and 1960s, a number of voluntary organizations developed to provide or lobby for improvements in services for disabled people. Special groups formed to help provide holidays for families of severely disabled people and to increase the level of mobility services, electronic devices, and income and benefits. Voluntary groups, such as the Disablement Income Group, developed to secure an income as a 'right' for disabled people. The large number of different benefits and different departments with separate responsibility for various services have made it difficult for disabled people to know about the services and benefits for which they are eligible and to follow the application procedures.

In the late 1960s, the increasing slowness in service provision by local authorities led to the establishment of a committee on personal social services, resulting in the 1968 Seebohm Report. This committee's review of personal, social, and allied services led to the recommendation that health and welfare services be separated, with the health service to be concerned with medical diagnosis and treatment and the welfare or social services departments to be concerned with other aspects of care such as social work, social rehabilitation, the provision of residential and day centres, home help, meals-on-wheels, holidays, aids to daily living, and adaptations to the homes of disabled people. This recommendation has been implemented through a series of legislative acts, including the National Health Service Act of 1984, which divorced health and welfare services completely.

Chronically Sick and Disabled Persons Act of 1970

The most important piece of legislation since 1948 has been the Chronically Sick and Disabled Persons Act of 1970 that made it mandatory for local authorities to identify and locate disabled people, determine their pressing needs, design or re-design services to help them, and inform them of existing services. By the time the act was published, it involved 11 ministeries and no less than 39 existing Acts of Parliament. This legislation, while not making specific mandatory provisions, encouraged local authorities to seek out disabled people and meet their needs.

Different sections of the 1970 Act provided for a wide number of services and policies that constitute a blueprint for service provision to disabled people. The provisions instituted by this legislation covered, for example, housing needs, meals-on-wheels and luncheon clubs, special housing and housing adaptions, legal access to public buildings including educational establishments, representation of the interests of disabled people, mobility aids, and the 'orange badge' disabled driver or passenger scheme. It is possible that the most important feature of the act was its success in publicizing the social needs and situation of disabled people to the broader community. Uneven implementation of the various provisions and its slow effect on subsequent legislation, however, have weakened some of the fundamental changes in social attitudes and social policy for disabled people (Topliss and Gould 1981).

The success of the 1970 legislation depended, as before, on the resources available to a particular local authority. New and improved services that require additional funds have not been implemented in some authorities, regardless of their wish to implement a 'charter' for disabled people and their families. Occupational therapists are the only professional workers employed by social services departments that are concerned exclusively with the provision of care for disabled people. The number of therapists so employed varies considerably. Development of their services depends on whether departmental heads and committees are sympathetic to the new demands of the 1970 Act, on the personalities and interests of occupational therapists in senior positions of influence, and on the relationships between managers and occupational therapists (Scrivens 1982). In departments that did not employ occupational therapists before 1970, social workers took on many of their tasks. Across the country there remains wide disparity in the extent of professional skills available to disabled clients.

Proposals for change

There are two main arguments in favour of changes in the methods by which government resources are allocated to disabled people. One argument is that the bifurcation of the allocative system into essentially an income maintenance system and a system for making in-kind provisions of goods and services, is unjustified. Financial problems, it is argued, are at the root of social disadvantage, and a unified system that concentrated upon cash allocations might better help recipients overcome disadvantage. An alternative view is that the two systems should remain separate because they fulfill different policy objectives, but greater fairness or equity is needed for the allocation of both cash and services.

Unifying the system

Arguments in favour of a unified system centre on a belief that the goals of the present methods of allocation are ill-conceived. Given the *ad hoc* way in which policies have developed, it is often difficult to identify precise goals, although a number of rationalizations have been offered. Richard Titmuss (1976), for example, described the social security system as 'distributive' as opposed to 're-distributive'. The main 'distributive' role is simply to ensure that everyone has a basic amount of money to meet immediate and future needs. The aim of the income maintenance system is therefore not to achieve a 'fair' redistribution of money in society, but to ensure that nobody is deprived of the basic necessities of life. In contrast, welfare services contain an element of rehabilita-tion in helping individuals overcome immediate and specific disabilities, often when an individual is not able to make the best decision concerning his or her own well-being.

One justification for providing services and goods instead of cash is the idea that financial poverty is not necessarily related to physical or social circumstances. Research studies have shown, however, that there is a cyclical relationship between chronic illness and low income (Buttler *et al.* 1981). Further evidence suggests that the problems of life for which in-kind provisions are made are concentrated in the lower occupational classes. Because it is difficult to distinguish between the effects of being in a low occupational group and the effects of a relative lack of money, it is possible to argue that increased income would alleviate many of the social problems experienced by such groups in society.

A fundamental division of opinion exists over how social inequalities should be overcome, and this division depends on how the causal relationship between poverty and disadvantage is perceived (Douglas 1976). Where the concern is to overcome disadvantage completely, the policy objective is to ensure that individuals consume enough to meet their basic needs, however these needs are defined. Consumption of goods and services is the most important policy consideration, and money transfers are justified only if it is felt that the free market will provide consumption more easily and at less cost than direct provision. Where the main concern is to decrease relative disadvantage, the policy objective is to ensure that everyone can participate freely in the market economy. The less well-off require money to express their wants and preferences in the market place. Quality of life is maintained, in this argument, not simply by the receipt or possession of goods and services, but by some intrinsic quality of the act of purchasing. To give goods and services directly denies the consumer the ability to exercise choice, and this can, over a lifetime, lead to a detrimental effect on the happiness and welfare of the individual. Thus, only money can ensure full participation in society.

If the main emphasis of social policy were placed upon income maintenance, professional welfare workers who are part of the income maintenance systems could provide assistance with the day-to-day problems experienced by 'socially disadvantaged' people. As in France, professional workers could be employed to specialize in the problems of specific groups whose income needs are clearly defined. Thus, disabled people who receive many transfers to help them with particular aspects of life could also receive personal services to help with their specific difficulties.

Although policy arguments in favour of in cash or in-kind allocations appear to be very different, the differences are more theoretical than practical. A system of cash allocations that made certain goods or services compulsory, such as education or health insurance, would achieve the same level of consumption as a direct in-kind system of provision. For the consumer, cash benefits would enhance the ability to choose among different types of goods and services, whereas with services the consumer is more limited to the monopoly of services delivered by the State.

Given the limited practical implications of the distinction between cash and in-kind allocations, it is hardly surprising that the debate has tended to concentrate on the final levels of benefit or service consumption rather than on the need to change organization and administrative systems. Consequently, the discussion has tended to emphasize the injustices or unfairness of the present system and to make recommendations for reducing the inequalities.

Increasing equity

As we have already discussed, disablement policies tend to develop as *ad hoc* responses to identified problems. As a result, there are great disparities not only in the type of benefits available, but also in the value of benefits for individuals with the same type and level of impairment. Marked regional variations exist in the availability as well as accessibility of services for disabled people. Many would argue that 'equal treatment for equal need' is the only fair social policy for disabled people. That is, all people in the same circumstances should have the right to receive services of the same quality, quantity, and type, which is the major principle of horizontal equality (Bebbington and Davies 1983). Similarly, greater resources should be made available to those in greater need, which is the major principle of vertical equity (West 1981).

The proposal for a comprehensive disability allowance or income, directed toward horizontal and vertical need, has been put forward by groups promoting the interests of disabled people. The Disability Alliance (1975) saw a three-fold policy objective in such a proposal:

(1) to distribute resources among disabled people so that those within equally severe disablement, irrespective of the cause or place of impairment, are entitled to similar weekly allowances or pensions;
(2) to bring the incomes of disabled people up to the level of non-disabled people;
(3) to eliminate poverty among disabled people.

To receive either financial assistance or services, a disabled client often faces a means test to establish entitlement to cash or to free or reduced payment for services. Means tests have been accused of deterring individuals from applying for benefits and services. In both cases, the anticipated numbers of applicants have proved higher than the actual number of people who have come forward. In 1970, researchers estimated that the home-help service would have to double to meet the demands of elderly citizens; (Hunt 1978). Similar findings were reported by a government survey to handicap (Harris 1971). Like the findings reported earlier for aids for daily living, disabled respondents in these surveys reported that they perceive a need for care that they have not translated into a demand for services. An analysis of the expressed needs or demands for either cash or services by disabled people involves different types of rationing.

Rationing

While resource allocation concerns the distribution of resources at an aggregate or program level, rationing refers to the process of distributing resources at more of an individual level. Allocation decisions usually set the constraints within which rationing occurs. Rationing systems reduce the demands for cash or services and, like allocation systems, come into operation before the consumer requests a provision (Scrivens, 1979).

There may well be insufficient resources to meet all the demands of those eligible to consume them. Hence, the rationing process constrains the demand for provision. Potential claimants may choose not to ask for help for many reasons. They may fear the possibility of acquiring a social stigma in the eyes of their friends or relatives, or they may feel demeaned by such dependency. More simply, disabled people may not know that they are entitled to help or may be ignorant of its existence. For example, the priorities study of preferences for cash or services among disabled people in Lambeth found that relatively few respondents had applied for services themselves (Scrivens and Caulfield 1983). Friends, relatives, or service workers with whom they were already in contact had approached the services for them. In addition, applying for some services can involve not only the expense of getting to the service but also other costs in terms of time that could have been used otherwise.

Rationing a service, therefore, is the process by which limited resources are divided among various individuals competing for them. Three types of rationing in the supply of services have been identified: primary, secondary, and tertiary (Scrivens, 1979).

Primary rationing is the dismissal of expressed demands for services that providers deem as unsuitable for treatment or that do not fall within the working definition of need. The income maintenance service can use primary rationing only, as financial aid is guaranteed to all those who are eligible for it, although the amount given is determined by standard allocation and eligibility criteria. Services, on the other hand, tend to be allocated according to a variety of principles, the majority of which are controlled by the fact that the resources are limited.

The availability of resources is determined by the nature of the commodity provided. A distinction must be drawn between stocks (provisions of a single 'one off' variety) and flows (provisions with a continuous nature). The former includes such items as aids to daily living. Only a limited number of aids are allocated at any one time and these do not require replacement for long periods. The latter includes service goods that are needed immediately and on a regular basis, such as home-help services or meals-on-wheels. Where stocks are involved, the availability of resources is dependent upon the total amount of resources available within a given time period. Flows, however, are a more flexible provision, and the amount received can be varied by reducing the amount of time spent with each client or by reducing the frequency of service delivery.

Primary rationing is the basis of the present provision system for services and financial benefits. Its objective is to sort out those eligible and ineligible to receive help. In the case of financial benefit, eligibility is determined primarily by rigid criteria based on a variety of principles that are well-defined for each benefit.

Services, on the other hand, are allocated on the basis of need as determined by professionals.

When demand exceeds supply, a common practice is to delay a response to acceptable demands until resources become available to meet them. The most common form of this resource rationing, which is known as secondary rationing, is the 'waiting list'. Even when the consumer finally receives a service, he or she can be faced with yet another form of rationing, known as tertiary rationing, in which the quality or quantity of the service provided to each individual is reduced to allow more people to receive resources. The amount of time devoted to a client and the quality of the provision may be reduced, for example. Also, a poor substitute for a service may be provided, such as appointing an inexperienced welfare officer to a particularly difficult case.

These different forms of rationing have led to demands for changes in the existing system of provision. Which changes are recommended depends on the sort of rationing that is causing the greatest concern. Where tertiary rationing occurs, often too few resources are available to meet the high demand for them. The quality of the provision will be diluted if the authorities provide less service, time, money, or material help to all individual clients, rather than turn some clients away. If the degree of dilution is too great, the goods or services may not benefit the client or may even cause harm. Secondary rationing, which causes people to wait for long periods of time before being treated, many cause unnecessary distress. Waiting lists exist for most adaptions and rehabilitation services provided by social services departments. In a study of the work of local authority occupational therapists, a number of therapists claimed that clients had to wait over a month to be seen for assessment (Scrivens 1982). In the Lambeth study, 3 per cent of the disabled sample in Phase I reported that they were waiting for an initial visit from the social services department of their local authority.

Critics of primary and secondary rationing tend to support the need for some form of primary rationing. If resource allocation is left to the discretion of the professional, primary rationing should work in theory as an efficient and just means of allocating resources. Universal access to the services is possible and the 'needy' are selected by the professional assessor. Those who do not demand the service, yet could benefit from it, obviously are a concern, but the main principle behind the provision of services is that access should be voluntary and disabled individuals should decide whether they wish to receive the service. Advocates of increased equity in the provision of services argue that if all people are equally at risk of requiring help from the services, then everybody should have the same opportunity to acquire them. Thus, services should be provided universally across the country and be designed for people to use them as necessary.

Of more concern to those promoting increased equity is the deprivation of resources among disabled people who do not meet precise eligibility requirements. If a broad definition of State-provided resources is taken, then the severely disabled who receive income from the State, as well as services and cash benefits, can receive disproportionately more than do moderately disabled people who do not receive income or choose to use services. This is a major policy problem in making homogeneous provisions for a population as diverse as disabled people. Not only do medical conditions and impairments differ enormously in their nature, but the effect of disablement on quality of life varies widely from person-to-person.

As shown in Chapters 2 and 4, the effect of using a broad definition of disability is to increase the number of people identified as disabled and increase the assessed severity of disability. Thus, a policy that is based on a broad definition of disability will expand the population eligible for help. If limited resources are available, those resources will have to be spread across even more people, and the rationing process becomes extended.

Response to the allocation system

Data from the Lambeth survey indicate that there is a large number of people with functional limitations for whom specific services that they perceive as beneficial are not available. Some people argue that there should be some compensation for this unmet need. However, devising and providing services to meet their specific needs is not practical or economically feasible. The major viable option is to make compensatory provision in cash, allowing disabled people to buy any services they need without recourse to local authority- or State-provided services.

The only practicable way to determine whether this idea is appealing to disabled people is to ask them. In Phase III of the Lambeth Health Survey, disabled respondents were asked whether they would like to receive more cash or more services. Table 7.3 illustrates their responses. Nearly twice as many disabled respondents who reported that they would like more help preferred cash benefits over services. The majority (56 per cent), however, felt they should not get any more help than they were already getting. This preference to maintain the status quo and not to take additional resources also was reflected in the priorities study, conducted specifically to establish the preferences of disabled people for cash or services (Scrivens and Caulfield 1983). Respondents were asked whether they would like to receive cash or services instead of their present levels of service receipt. The majority chose to receive what they were already getting and rejected the idea of change. Even those who were not receiving services chose to get nothing rather than to take cash compensation for their lack of services. It would appear, therefore, that the majority of disabled people interviewed in both studies felt that the present allocation system was not only acceptable but also fair. The system that disabled people are used to is the one that they understand, and respondents appeared to be satisfied with the present system.

While disabled people appear to find it difficult to envisage a

Table 7.3. *Preferences for cash benefits of services among disabled respondents*

Statement or question	Number and (proportion) of disabled respondents			
	Agree	Disagree	Can't say	N
Government should give more help to disabled people in general	482 (81)	86 (14)	28 (5)	596 (100)
I, personally, should receive more help	227 (38)	334 (56)	25 (4)	596 (100)
If agree, would you prefer *more cash?*	172 (76)	48 (20)	10 (4)	227 (100)

change in the existing system of provision, fairness in a democratic society calls for tapping the opinions of non-disabled people. Taxpayers provide the means for provision and their votes are important to making choices. When non-disabled respondents in the Lambeth Health Survey were asked whether disabled people should get more help of any kind from the State, the majority (81 per cent) reported that they should. Likewise, the same majority of *disabled* respondents thought disabled people in general should get more help, although they themselves felt no need for more help (See Table 7.3). This finding suggests a discrepancy between people's perceptions of their own conditions and needs and those of others.

Toward universal benefit

A fundamental conflict remains between two different principles for the allocation of State resources to disabled people. One principle is concerned with concentrating resources on those who need them most. The other is concerned with compensating disabled people not only for the misfortunes experienced due to their disablement and the relative decrease in the quality of their lives, but also for the extra financial and welfare needs they incur.

If a truly equitable system was introduced, with equal treatment for equal need, it would be necessary to compensate those who could not benefit from or receive available services for one reason or another. The only feasible way of achieving this objective is to produce cash, although the implications for the allocation system would be dramatic. Cash, on the other hand, has universal application and could be appreciated by those who do not want services.

Determining who should receive such compensation would require complex regulations controlling eligibility in order to maintain fairness. In addition, the criteria probably would have to be defined very stringently to limit the population to whom help is given and to restrict the consumption of resources. Second, strict criteria are needed to ensure that only those who deserve help, based on the definition of eligibility, actually receive it. As the Lambeth study shows, the wider the definition of disability, the more people there are who will fit the criteria and be entitled to receive resources.

The present allocation is undoubtedly unjust from a number of theoretical viewpoints. It would seem, however, that the present system at least has evolved a set of allocative criteria that work, are affordable, and are acceptable to society at large and, more importantly, to disabled people. Movements toward changing the system are more likely to occur through the incremental expansion of the population of disabled people who are entitled to receive income benefits, as demonstrated by recent policy innovations such as the Housewives' Non-Contributory Invalidity Pension. To revise the present system substantially would prove complex. Continuing debate through research and experimentation may improve the less satisfactory elements of the provision for cash and services.

References

Bebbington, A. C. and Davis, B. (1983). Equality and efficiency in the allocation of the personal social services. *Journal of Social Policy* **12**, 309–30.

Beveridge, W. (1942). *Social insurance and allied services*. Cmnd 6502. HMSO, London.

Buttler, L. W., Neewacket P. W., Piontkowski, D. L., Harper A. K., and Franks, P. E. (1981). *Low income and illness: an analysis of national health policy and the poor*. School of Medicine, University of California, San Francisco.

Disability Alliance. (1975). *Poverty and disability. The case for a comprehensive income scheme for disabled people*. The Disability Alliance, London.

Douglas, M. (1976). Relative poverty—relative communication. In *Traditions in social policy: essays in honour of Violet Buttler*. (ed A. H. Hackney). Basil Blackwell, Oxford.

Harris, A. I. (1971). *The handicapped and impaired in Great Britain*. HMSO, London.

Hunt, A. (1978). *The Elderly at Home*. London, HMSO.

Keeble, U. (1979). *Aids and adaptations: occupational papers on social administration*. Bedford Square Press, London.

Manpower Services Commission (1981). *Review of the quota scheme for the employment of disabled people*. Manpower Services Commission, London.

Scrivens, E. (1979). Towards a theory of rationing. *Social Policy and Administration* **13**, 53–64.

Scrivens, E. (1982). Rationing theory and practice. *Social Policy and Administration* **16**, 136–48.

Scrivens, E. and Caulfield B. (1983). *Report of a pilot study to investigate consumer preference for cash or services.* DHSS, London.

Simpkins, J. (1978). *Whose benefit?* Disablement Income Group, London.

Titmuss, R. M. (1976). *Commitment of welfare.* George Allen and Unwin, London.

Topliss, E. (1982). *Social responses to handicaps.* Longman Group Limited, London.

Topliss, E. and Gould, B. (1981) *Charter for the disabled.* Basil Blackwell and Martin Robertson, Oxford.

West, P. A. (1981). Equity and efficiency in the national health service in England. *Social Science and Medicine.* **15**, 117–22.

8

Income, work, and disability

PETER WEST

> Work, for many of us, is the way we meet the people we most
> esteem and cherish. Work is what distracts us, at times for
> weeks on end, from life's incessant chaos and uncertainty.
> Even when it is menial, as everybody's often is, work confers
> some degree of pattern, purpose, and continuity. It is, as
> Sigmund Freud declared, one of the two really big things in
> life, and of the two it is by far the most likely to be there when
> you need it. Its seeds can be sown long before the beginning
> of parenthetical 'careers', and its blooms, with a little luck
> and attention, can be perennial.
>
> Jane Howard

A major element governing the welfare of disabled people is
income. While financial independence may never fully offset the
loss of activities due to disablement, it can provide alternatives to
those activities. Having a car, for example, can take the place of
walking distances, or the home may be modified for greater
convenience. This chapter examines the relationship between
disability and income in the labour market and the implications for
special employment and income support policies provided for
disabled people by the central government. The labour market,
the major source of income for most households, is considered
first. Subsequent sections examine the principles that underlie
employment opportunities for disabled workers and income
support provided by social security. The extent to which the labour
market can accommodate special employment provisions and
income support for disabled people is also discussed.

Disability and the labour market

The labour market functions, albeit with manifold imperfections,
as a mechanism for matching demand for labour with the supply of

various skills in various locations. An employer hires an individual, believing that the person has the ability to do the job, or is the best choice for the wages offered. Thus, each job is a test of ability across a spectrum of skills. For many jobs, however, the range of skills may be relatively narrow. Moreover, given the indoor, sedentary nature of most clerical work and the limited mobility and physical strength required for much industrial work, many physical disabilities should not preclude employment. In fact, most employers consider a capacity for mental and manual work to be much more important than mobility or physical agility.

But mobility can be an important factor in determining whether disabled individuals are employed. While they may possess all the skills needed for a job, their chances of being employed may be reduced simply by not being able to get to work or to travel in search of a job. Their chances for employment, or their wages, will also be reduced if the employer must modify the work place without receiving a subsidy. Similarly, certain physical restrictions may force many skilled disabled people to retire prematurely. Consequently, being disabled may prevent people from competing on equal terms with other workers, even though they may possess the necessary skills.

Unemployment among disabled people is often a reflection of supply difficulties, such as inability to travel to work or to offer the right skills. However, it may also be caused by demand problems, such as the need to modify the work place, or by discrimination on the part of the employer. It is difficult to determine how much supply and demand problems each contribute to the unemployment of disabled people. In examining the data from community surveys, we cannot conclude whether it is poor access to work, lack of appropriate skills, reluctance to hire due to additional costs, or plain discrimination that is reducing employment opportunities. Data from the Lambeth study show only the consequences of an active labour market for disabled people of working age.

The following analysis, based on the Lambeth study, focuses in particular on men of working age, since the open market is the primary source of income for this group, as opposed to women or people past retirement age whose income is based on their working history. The Lambeth survey did not address the lifetime profile of disability, thus precluding an adequate analysis of retirement income. However, the principles or objectives behind

Table 8.1. *Working status of men at first interview*

Working status	Disabled men (%)	Controls (%)
Employed	58	86
Unemployed	10	4
Retired	10	0
Chronic sick	17	0
Student	1	7
N	279	102

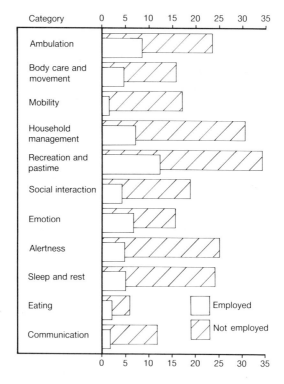

Fig. 8.1. Functional Limitations Profile for disabled men under 65: employed compared with not employed. Mean dysfunction score standardized so that maximum possible dysfunction score = 100.

an income policy for young disabled people probably apply just as well to women and retired disabled people. Both those past retirement age and those excluded from work due to disability— no matter what their age or sex—must rely on sources of income outside the labour market. The State, in particular, is required to provide both groups with sufficient funds for a minimum standard of living.

The exclusion of women from the empirical analysis here is a consequence of the greater heterogeneity of labour market activity by women. Some women who remain employed have income profiles similar to those of male colleagues. For many women, however, the social pressures or voluntary decision to work within the home restricts or curtails their employment. In general, female employment is characterized by extensive part-time working, limited job search, and wages below those of men. Involuntary and voluntary absence from the labour market leaves many women with no direct personal income. Consequently, assessing the impact of physical disability on income is more complex for women than for men. However, considering policy commitment and limited legislative progress towards equality of earning opportunities for women, disabled women should benefit from policy initiatives designed to improve the welfare of their male counterparts.

Disability and employment

The disadvantages that disabled men face in competing for jobs are shown by their lower rates of employment. In each age group, disabled men at Phase I of the Lambeth study had lower employment rates than did the controls, as demonstrated by the combined working-age groups in Table 8.1.

Unemployment, early retirement, and chronic sickness were correspondingly higher for disabled people. Not surprisingly, the unemployed disabled men had a higher FLP score than those in employment (Fig. 8.1). Thirty per cent of disabled respondents linked their unemployment or retirement to health problems. The difficulty of travelling to work was the most frequently cited problem (21 per cent), but almost the same proportion of the disabled respondents (20 per cent) felt that employers discriminated against them.

Disabled people who are working may suffer loss of income or job prospects because they need to change aspects of their work to cope with health problems. Ten per cent of disabled workers were working shorter hours due to their health, and 16 per cent were restricted to light work. However, the limited extent to which disabilities hinder the performance of a specific job is illustrated by the fact that the majority of the disabled respondents were employed and reported no particular restrictions in their work. This finding may mean that this group of respondents has not suffered any disadvantages at work due to their disabilities. Equally, it could be that the diversity of jobs available and the actions of employees and employers are sufficient to ensure that individuals with a range of functional limitations are channelled into work where their disability does not affect performance at work, their access to work, or at least their perceptions of them. Since there is no way that such channelling would direct workers to higher-paid jobs, directing disabled workers in this way is likely to lead to lower incomes.

Disability and income

As a result of reduced employment opportunities, disabled people have lower incomes than other people. Consequently, they are largely dependent on social security payments from the State, which are likely to be insufficient to raise their income to the higher levels enjoyed by most employed people.

The lower incomes of disabled people have been reported by a number of social surveys (e.g. Townsend 1979; Sainsbury 1970). Comparisons between different surveys are complicated by different definitions of disability, different income ranges, and the effects of inflation and rising unemployment. However, while disabled people have received large compensations in a few well-publicized cases, the preponderance of the evidence shows that disabled people are generally poorer than most people, as we would expect from their disadvantages in the labour market.

Income data from Phase I of the Lambeth survey are reported in Table 8.2. Forty eight per cent of disabled men are in the bottom two income groups, compared with 33 per cent of other men. While these figures highlight the disproportionate relationship between disability and income, they also show that disability is not the only influence on income. Appreciable numbers of men without a disability reported low incomes. This finding reflects the innate operation of the labour market, that is, the pursuit of the right skills at the right price in the right place.

Table 8.2. *Proportion of disabled and control male respondents by level of income at first interview*

Income per week (£)	Disabled persons (%)	Non-disabled persons (%)
Less than 25	19	12
25–40	29	21
40–55	14	14
55–70	16	21
70–85	6	12
85–100	6	9
100–120	2	2
120–140	2	3
Greater than 140	1	1
Not answered	6	5
N	395	146

As a consequence of the uncertainty of the labour market, those without disability may nonetheless find themselves relatively disadvantaged. Thus, as far as income support policy is concerned, there is no clear separation between the poor with or without specific disabilities, other than accounting for the high cost of living faced by some disabled people. Both groups suffer disadvantages from being without work or being channelled into low-paying jobs.

As expected, the lower employment rate for disabled men in the sample contributes appreciably to their lower incomes. The analyzed income data from the Lambeth survey showed that it is the interaction of disability and the labour market that is most important. Unemployment and inability to work due to poor health were closely related to low income in the sample. The degree of disability had much less impact on income because, as noted earlier, the FLP reflects a wider range of disability than would prevent a disabled person from participating in the labour market.

Employment policy

If the disadvantages of disabled workers in the labour market lead to reduced employment and income, social policy can seek to improve their positions by changing the market environment or by providing income support measures. The Manpower Services Commission (1978) has much of the responsibility for improving the employment opportunities for disabled men and women. The options open to it are concerned predominantly with changing the demands for disabled workers in the marketplace. This can be done by changing employers' perceptions of disabled workers, removing barriers to employment, subsidizing employment, or creating employment.

Current policy includes commitments to orient more employers to disabled workers and to promote job introduction schemes in which disabled people are employed on a trial basis. Barriers to the employment of disabled people, such as the need to modify the work place or the work task, can be overcome to a degree by using public funds to pay for modifications. New capital grants are to be offered for this purpose. Subsidization of disabled workers is not favoured for several reasons, one of which is the risk of creating a pool of 'cheap' disabled labour. The employer can take on such labour at rates effectively below those for able-bodied people, with the subsidy from the State making up the difference. Finally, there is a commitment in current policy to raise the number of places for sheltered employment, which essentially is a work place operated by the State.

There will always be a need to educate and encourage employers to hire disabled workers, if only because of basic prejudices against disabled people. Grants to modify the work place may be less useful for a number of reasons. The disabled work force is not homogeneous. There are a number of general disabilities associated with impairments in the body's major systems, such as chest disease, heart disease, and mental disorders (see Chapter 5). These are not likely to be directly affected by modifications to the work task, although in some cases the purchase of specific equipment may help the disabled worker. For example, lifting equipment will reduce the strain on the heart and lungs of a warehouseman. The direct modification of a job is more likely to be useful for a worker with a specific disability, such as a missing limb or blindness. Modifying the task may also have the disadvantage of making it specific to a particular kind of disability. Even where this is not the case, the employer may perceive it as a narrowing of his future choice of employees.

Subsidy raises the possibility of friction with other workers and claims of cheap labour. Of course, subsidies have been widely established in policies for increasing the employment of other disadvantaged groups, such as unemployed young people. Not surprisingly, claims of cheap labour have been directed at these subsidies too.

Sheltered employment may provide jobs in a supportive environment for workers whose disabilities would otherwise prevent employment. But in some cases, such work may be stigmatizing because it lumps disabled workers together, sometimes doing relatively unskilled work, and is not regarded as 'real' work by disabled people seeking employment without segregation.

The heterogeneity of disabled people seeking work is illustrated by the breakdown of the diseases suffered by people on the disabled register, although some disabled people seeking work probably do not register. Diseases and injuries of limbs and of the spine affect more than 30 per cent of registered people. The remaining 70 per cent fall into 16 other diagnostic categories, none of which accounts for more than 11 per cent of all registered people. These diseases, such as circulatory disease (11 per cent of registered disabled people), chest disease (8 per cent), and arthritis (4.5 per cent), are essentially chronic and degenerative. This fact could discourage employers by reducing their confidence in the ability of the worker to attend work regularly. More generally, disabled men and women of working age are highly heterogeneous in the mix of their skills. Consequently, a flexible approach will inevitably be required to identify and overcome the diverse problems they face in securing employment.

Income replacement for disabled people

Income support policy determines the income level for many disabled people, since they have less employment opportunities and must rely on social security. From the standpoint of market economics, the reference level of income for disabled people is the amount they could command if they were able-bodied. Any income policy must therefore take account of how much income is generated by the labour market and how it is distributed among the population. The main question then becomes: For a disabled man or women no longer employed, what is an appropriate income level against which income support should be determined independent of other payments for a disabled person's higher cost of living? Without knowing what the person would earn without disability, there is no clear reference income. Policy-makers must therefore decide where a particular disabled person should stand in the income distribution compared with skilled and unskilled workers. If the disabled person previously worked, past income provides a reference point. In this case, the policy dilemma is whether to pay past level of income from public funds.

While it is entirely legitimate to restore the standard of living lost because of disability, disabled people compete for public funds with other disadvantaged groups such as pensioners, the unemployed, and those in poverty due to family size or circumstances. Providing a higher income for a group from fixed tax revenue, simply because its members were previously in well-paid jobs, conflicts with the provision of a more modest increase for the wider group of recipients, even though disabled people probably rank high in receiving public sympathy.

At present, income support for disabled people is provided through a wide range of benefits in Great Britain and abroad. Each benefit is assessed according to particular eligibility criteria, and the matching of a given set of system, which has arisen through piecemeal change, is related to the concepts of impairment, disability, and handicap, each of which would provide a different basis for income support.

Impairment as a criterion for income support is akin to a system of insurance compensation whereby individual bodily parts are valued and payment is made for their loss. Under such a system, the State would give every person suffering the loss of a leg the same level of income.

Income support based on disability, the loss of activity due to the impairment, would discriminate against those who in some way overcome their restriction. Fitter or more determined people may almost completely replace activities lost from loosing a leg by using prostheses, for example. Their disability is lessened, thereby reducing their entitlement to income support.

Handicap is even more complicated as a basis for income support because of the subtle interactions of disabled people and their environments. An amateur sportsman may suffer appreciably if a sporting injury prevents further participation, even though he may still be fitter than average. On the other hand, a highely-paid professional sportsman similarly injured could receive appreciable insurance compensation for his or her loss. As noted earlier in this chapter, financial security may permit adjustments in lifestyle and environment that somewhat reduce the handicap. However, it would take a very subtle policy indeed to discern all the effects of handicap, considering the ultimate psychic burden on the individual.

In view of the difficulty of assessing handicap, there is perhaps some merit in the current income support policy, which offers to replace income lost from work and provides a number of specific payments to those with more easily identified impairments and disabilities. Mobility allowance, for example, provides financial support for those obviously restricted in getting around. Attendance allowance is payable to those who require round-the-clock support. One criticism of the present policy is that, with the myriad of available benefits, it is difficult to ensure that benefits have been offered to all eligible recipients. Consequently, some needs go unmet.

Policy is also complicated by the possible conflict between compensation for handicap and payment for disabled people's higher costs of living. The latter issue addresses the expenses incurred by handicapped people to attain a certain minimum standard of living or comfort, rather than compensating them for lost activities. For example, the reduced mobility of many disabled people keeps them at home most of the time. Therefore, they must heat their homes for longer periods of time at a higher cost. Although only one of many possible extra living costs, heating for disabled and elderly people has been a particular concern in recent years due to the rising cost of energy. Policy intervention has resulted to provide support for these extra living expenses, adding to the complexity of income support programmes.

A frequently proposed alternative system is the unified disability benefit, which is free of any qualification based on social security contributions in past employment. It would be paid to all disabled people, according to an assessment of the disability. It is not clear whether impairment or disability should be the standard for assessment. A drawback of both is that their link with handicap is not straightforward. Payments based on impairment would be independent of the income of recipients. Those able to secure well-paid employment would be treated identically to those who could not work.

The difficulty facing policy-makers is that income support funds for disabled people are inevitably below the level that many pressure groups regard as satisfactory. Without funding for a high, general disability benefit, there will be some pressure to pay less to those not suffering financial hardships, whatever their disability, even though well-paid disabled workers could repay a part of the benefit in taxation. One group of people who will be discriminated against in this process is those receiving financial compensation for disability through insurance companies or employers. Some people would view receipt of a public benefit as double payment for the disability.

From that viewpoint, it is a short step to discrimination against those who receive a high income from employment or assets, in spite of their disability. Limited funding may then lead to the use of means-tested benefits in order to concentrate on giving funds to the disabled poor, even though their disabilities may not be the sole source of their low incomes. Similarly, partitioning of benefits for specific needs appears attractive again as a method of channelling the maximum resources to the most needy, where need is a consequence of a variety of circumstances and not merely disability.

Finally, policy must address the link between disability and aging. Handicap can be assessed according to a normal range of activities of daily living, but the norm will clearly change for different age groups. Elderly people unable to undertake certain activities are not differentiated from most of their age cohort and so they are not considered disabled. Yet, relative to the young, they manifestly are disabled. If disability in old age is linked to the norm for the age group, we might expect to see disabled people lose their income support as they grow old and become less different from the average of their age cohort. On the other hand, if disability is viewed independent of age, income support to the old would rise with general loss of abilities by the cohort as a whole. While this system would be acceptable to many as a method of improving the quality of old age, younger employed groups would face higher taxes if significant payments were made for disability. A potentially higher tax rate for the young employed is unlikely to commend such a scheme to governments concerned about maintaining taxation at its present levels. On the other hand, it would do much to relieve the financial and psychic pressures of aging and disability for the elderly and others outside the work force.

Conclusion

The incomes of disabled people are undoubtedly depressed by their reduced employment, as confirmed by numerous social surveys. Policy for income support for disabled people is complicated by historical inequality in income distribution. This variation tends to lead to income support being directed at the lowest income group, despite the merits of an individual's claim to additional support or the cause of low income. The use of impairment, disability, or handicap as the standard for income support is also difficult to resolve. Finally, aging and disability are inevitably linked, and policy needs to reconsider how income support for the two can be made consistent. While a unified disability benefit has much to recommend it, the possible complexity and tax cost are likely to assure the continuance of the current fragmented system of benefits to the detriment of many disabled people.

References

Manpower Services Commission (1978). *Developing employment and training services for disabled people*. Management Services Commission, London.

Sainsbury, S. (1970). *Registered as disabled*. Occasional papers on social administration, No. 35. Bell, London.

Townsend, P. (1979). *Poverty in the United Kingdom*. Pelican Books, London.

9

Social ties, support, and well-being

MYFANWY MORGAN

> It is because society, weak and disturbed, lets too many persons escape too completely from its influence. Thus, the only remedy for the ill is to restore enough consistency to social groups for them to obtain a firmer grip on the individual, and for him to feel himself bound to them.

> Emile Durkheim, *Suicide*, 1897 (trans. 1951)

Relationships with kin, friends, and casual acquaintances form an important source of social support. This support can be divided broadly into instrumental aid, including financial and practical assistance, advice, and information, and socio-emotional aid consisting of affection, sympathy, understanding, and esteem (Kaplan *et al.* 1977).

Traditionally, attention has been focused on the role of social ties in providing instrumental aid, especially in caring for elderly and chronically ill people. It was widely believed prior to Harris' National Survey (1971) that this caring role had been largely taken over by the formal services. However, Harris' study (1971) and subsequent disability surveys have revealed that a large number of disabled people live in private households and obtain assistance with self-care tasks largely from relatives inside and outside the household. Only a small proportion of even the most severely disabled people receive domiciliary services on a regular basis. Disabled people in Lambeth received more services than those studied in Harris' National Survey, but only 16 per cent of them who were aged 45–75 and were classified as having a high level of physical disability (score of 35 or over) received meals on wheels in the last 14 days, only 26 per cent a home help, and only 10 per cent a visit from a district nurse.

The increasing proportion of elderly people aged 75 and over in the British population means there will be a growing number of chronically ill people requiring assistance and care. Caring for a severely disabled person, however, often places considerable burdens on the main carer and their family, including physical and mental strain, and in many cases, a need to give up paid employment. In addition, family activities may be restricted, generating more tension (Nissel and Bonnerjea 1982). Recognition of the social costs of caring for a severely dependent relative has led to a greater emphasis on the need for formal services, not only to replace informal assistance for those who lack close relatives, but also to act in partnership with the informal carers to reduce their burden of care (Walker 1987). However, it is important to note that the recent broadening of definitions of disability means that many people now classified as disabled require only limited assistance with self-care tasks. For example, of the 702 disabled respondents aged 25–75 who were interviewed in the second phase of the Lambeth survey, only 2 per cent had difficulty with feeding and 7 per cent with combing and brushing their hair (women) or shaving (men).

Informal support not only reduces needs for formal services by providing practical assistance and care, but may also exert a direct effect on health and feelings of well-being. This chapter reviews evidence of the general relationship between social ties and health and, using data from the Lambeth survey, examines the relationship between the availability of support and the physical and psychosocial functioning of disabled people.

The relationship between social ties and health

Durkheim's classic study of suicide (1897) provides the earliest systematic investigation and theoretical statement of the relationship between social ties and health. Durkheim suggested that suicide rates were high among those who were insufficiently integrated into society, and explained the higher suicide rate among Protestants than Roman Catholics, and unmarried compared with married people, to be due to the greater degree of integration of their respective religious and domestic groups. However, he also noted that an overly high level of integration and identification with social groups could increase risks of suicide. The ecological school during the 1930s and 1940s was also important in drawing attention to the relationship between the social disorganization of inner city areas, including the disruption of social ties, and mental illness (e.g. Faris and Dunham 1939). For a long period, however, the relationship between support and health was relatively neglected. Instead, epidemiological studies aimed to identify single or multiple risk factors for specific conditions. An important change in emphasis occurred from the 1970s, with the increasing acceptance of the view that differences in rates of morbidity and mortality between marital groups or social classes may be due to differences in their general susceptibility to disease (Najman 1980; Kasl 1982). The experience of stress was identified as an important vulnerability factor increasing risks of morbidity from a wide range of conditions through its effect on neural, hormonal, and immunological control systems, while the availability of support was regarded as an important protective factor, frequently serving to moderate the effects of stress. Studies providing evidence of the relationship between support and health can be broadly divided into survival studies and those examining the relationship between support and stress.

Survival studies

These studies follow a group of people over time and examine the relationship between the initial level of support given and subsequent changes in health or mortality rates. The most notable survival study to date is Berkman and Syme's (1979) 9-year follow-up of a random sample of nearly 7,000 adults aged 30–69 who were living in Alameda County, California. At the start of the survey, information on four sources of social contact was collected: marriage, contacts with close friends and relatives, church membership, and informal and formal group associations. Age and sex-specific mortality rates calculated for the 9-year period showed that respondents with each type of social tie had lower mortality rates than respondents lacking such connections. However, the more intimate ties of marriage and contacts with friends and relatives were stronger predictors of reduced mortality than were the ties of church and group membership. The age-adjusted mortality rate was more than twice as high for the most isolated group of men than for those with a large number of social connections, while for women the rate was nearly three times as high. Furthermore, when all four types of social contact were combined to form a Social Network Index (SNI), the relative risks associated with a low rank on the SNI were greater than those of any single network measure. To examine whether these findings were due to an association between the level of social connection and health status at the start of the study, people were classified into four health groups. For each category of physical health state, higher mortality rates remained among people with fewer social connections. The age-adjusted relative risks for mortality for persons with a low SNI varied, however, from 1.5 for people with no health problems to 3.5 among people classified as disabled. Berkman and Syme's study thus suggests that social contact may be especially important in determining the life expectations of people with chronic illness and disability. However, as the authors acknowledge, it is difficult to be sure that social ties are affecting health and that health has not had a prior selective effect in determining people's levels of social contact.

Social ties and life events

An important question is whether support exerts a protective effect through reducing the adverse health effects of stress. This has been examined in studies of people who have experienced a particular stressful life event, such as widowhood (Walker *et al.* 1977), unemployment or work stress (Gore 1978; Holohan and Moos 1981), and pregnancy (Nuckolls *et al.* 1972). In each case, people are classified by level of support, and the health experience of groups with different levels of support are compared.

In a 2-year follow-up study, for example, Gore (1978) investigated the physical and mental health consequences of involuntary job loss among a sample of 100 men. The men were classified on a 13-item index of social support that focused on their relationships and social activities with their wife (if present), relatives, and friends. Men in the lowest population tertile on this measure were designated as 'unsupported', and the others as 'supported'. Examination of the experiences of these groups revealed no differences between the unsupported and supported men with respect to weeks unemployed or actual economic deprivation. While unemployed, however, the unsupported men reported more physical complaints, had higher scores on an index of depression, and showed marked physiological changes, such as higher serum cholesterol concentrations.

The general conclusion drawn from Gore's study and many similar ones is that social ties exert a protective effect on health among people experiencing life changes. Such studies say nothing, however, about whether support exerts a protective effect on health *only* among people suffering the stressful effects of specific life events (buffering effect), or whether support also has a direct protective effect in the absence of life events, by for example, protecting the individual from the adverse effects of long-term life stresses and promoting healthy lifestyles (main effect).

The protective effect of support on health, both in the presence and absence of life events, is generally examined by comparing the relationship between the levels of support and health among two groups of people—those classified as experiencing a life event and those not experiencing such an event. In some cases, researchers have concluded that support has a protective effect on health, especially psychiatric states, irrespective of the presence of life events (Andrews *et al.* 1978; Williams *et al.* 1981). More commonly, the results are regarded as providing evidence of a buffering effect, since support has a greater effect on health among those experiencing life events (Linn *et al.* 1979; La Rocco *et al.* 1980). For example, Brown and Harris' (1978) study of the risks of depression among women showed that 10 per cent of women who experienced a severe event or major difficulty, but who enjoyed an intimate and confiding relationship with a husband or boyfriend (high support), developed depression compared with 32 per cent of women who experienced a severe event and lacked this form of supportive relationship. Among women who did not experience a severe event, one per cent with an intimate confiding relationship developed depression compared with three per cent lacking this strong social tie.

Findings concerning the relationship between support and health are influenced by the measures of support, life events, and health outcomes employed, as well as the population and time period studied (Thoits 1982; Cohen and Syme 1985). Support, for example, has been measured in terms of the size and composition of individual networks, including ties with kin and friends and social participation in groups and organizations, as well as by measures of the availability and strength of confiding relationships.

Similarly, life events are sometimes equated with undesirable life changes or life 'crises' which are viewed as stressful because of the loss they entail. Alternatively, the concept of life events can be broadened to include both undesirable and desirable events (e.g., marriage, job promotion), based on the belief that all change is stressful, requiring adaption to a changed situation, which can be wearing in itself as well as making people vulnerable to other stresses. Assessment of the stressfulness of events is sometimes determined by reference to weights derived from subjective scaling experiments, such as the Holmes–Rahe scale (1967) or one of its many modifications. An alternative approach is to assess the subjective meaning of events for the individual, as with Brown and Harris' (1978) use of independent observers to rate the undesirability of events in terms, for example, of the degree of threat and unpleasantness of the event, and whether it posed a long- or short-term threat, by eliciting the respondents own feelings and responses. These differences emphasize the importance of relating findings of the association between support and health to the measures and populations studied.

Support and well-being in the Lambeth study

Whereas most studies focus on the onset of illness, the Lambeth study examined the relationship between the level of support and changes in functioning during the course of illness. A 2-year 'survival' study was undertaken to examine the relationship between respondents' level of support at the first interview and their risks of mortality and changes in physical and psychosocial scores as recorded at the third interview. Support was measured in terms of social contact, with an overall score derived from five sources of social contact (Fig. 9.1). Respondents were classified into high and low levels of social contact because contact scores may not form a ratio scale, that is, twice the contact does not necessarily imply twice the support. However, the high and low groups distinguished broad differences in levels of support.

Between the first and third interviews of the Lambeth study, 47 deaths were recorded among disabled people over the age of 25. Although this is a small number of deaths, the disabled people who died were more likely to have had a low level of social support (72 per cent) compared with the survivors (49 per cent), a finding

Social contact
This composite measure was based on five sources of social contact:
household size; people outside the household seen regularly; full- or
part-time employment; contact with selected health and social services
(home help, district nurse, meals on wheels, luncheon club, or day
centre); and attendance at church or religious groups. (Participation in
social activities outside the home was also included in Phase III.)

Points were assigned to each type of contact: Full-time work
received a higher score than part-time work, and the score for
household members varied according to the number of people in the
household. The scores for individual sources of social contact were
summed to provide an overall score.

Network emotional support
Respondents were asked whether they would confide in each of the
members of their personal network, which was defined as including up
to 20 people. The number of people in whom the respondents would
confide provides an overall network support score.

Loneliness (Phase II only)
Respondents were asked if they ever felt lonely, and if so, whether
they felt lonely all or most of the time, or a little of the time, or
whether they never felt lonely.

Main confiding relationship (Phase III only)
Respondents were asked who they would most likely turn to if they
wanted advice or reassurance. Second, they were asked whether they
would confide in this person about each of five problems, and third,
whether they would expect their main confidant to confide in them
about these sorts of problems. On the basis of their answers,
respondents were assigned a score ranging from 0 (no main confidant)
to 6 (confidant satisfies each dimension of confiding).

Fig. 9.1. Social support as measured in the Lambeth Health Survey.

supported by previous work. However, the deceased also had
significantly higher FLP scores; 60 per cent had a score of 20 or
more, compared with 27 per cent for the survivors. In addition,
they were more likely to be male (60 per cent compared with 42
per cent), or elderly (60 per cent over 65-years-old compared with
33 per cent under that age).

A particular problem in examining the influence of support on changes in functioning among disabled people is that many chronic conditions, such as arthritis and depression, are subject to fluctuations. The relationship between the level of support and 'steady deterioration' was therefore examined to identify people who were likely to have experienced a long-term decline in functioning rather than merely a series a fluctuations (see note in Table 9.1 and Chapter 4). The analysis was based on 494 respondents aged 45–75 who were interviewed in each of the three phases of the survey (85 per cent retention of Phase I sample). The relationship between the level of support at the first interview and the probability of being a 'deteriorator' was examined, controlling not only for the age and sex of respondents, but also for initial level of disability. Initial level of disability was included in the regression analysis to take account of the association between level of support and disability at the first interview, thus reducing the possibility that any observed association between level of support and health might be due to differences in health of the low- and high-support groups.

Slightly more than 20 per cent of respondents were classified as

Table 9.1. *Regression analysis of probability of being a 'deteriorator' in the Lambeth Health Survey by level of support (controlling for age, sex, and initial level of functioning)*

Initial level of social contact (1)	Physical deterioration	Psychosocial deterioration
High (score over 30) N = 222	0.25	0.27
Low (score 0–30) N = 272	0.30	0.36*

* p < .05 comparing high and low levels of social contact
Physical score consists of items relating to ambulation, mobility, body care and movement, and household management. Psychosocial score consists of items relating to emotion, alertness, sleep and rest, recreation, and social interaction.
Steady deterioration in functioning was defined as an increase in physical or psychosocial score by five units or more between first and third interviews, and the second interview score did not lie more than six units below the first interview value.
(1) Based on five-item measure of social contact (Fig. 9.1)

deteriorators in each of the categories of physical and psychosocial functioning. Respondents with a low level of support were more likely to deteriorate in both physical and psychosocial functioning than those with a high level of support, although the difference between support groups was statistically significant only for psychosocial functioning (Table 9.1). This finding, together with the higher mortality rate of the low support group, thus provides evidence of a positive relationship between support and health.

A further analysis was undertaken to determine the relationship between support and changes in functioning in the presence and absence of life events. This was based on 583 disabled people, aged 45–75, who were interviewed in the first two phases of the study. Respondents were asked at the second interview about their life events during the previous 12 months, using the following open-ended question:

Some people find that major events in their lives can have an effect on their general well-being. Since we last saw you a year ago, has anything happened which you feel has greatly changed your life?

Respondents were left to volunteer information they considered relevant. This method was adopted instead of providing a list of events for respondents to check, in the belief that an open-ended question would encourage respondents to report events that had a particular significance to them. All responses that did not concern the respondent's own health were recorded and coded into three categories: positive (generally desirable events); adverse (generally undesirable events); or ambiguous (desirability unclear as strongly influenced by individual perceptions and circumstances—for example, changed job, son or daughter left home). Since the focus of the study was on the effects of life crises, adverse events were chosen as the measure of life events. The most common adverse events reported were the death of a spouse or close family member, a major illness in the family, a major financial difficulty, and unemployment. Sixty-four respondents (11 per cent) reported one or more such adverse life events. This small number is comparable to the findings of other general population studies (Goldberg and Comstock 1980). The study may have slightly underestimated the occurrence of adverse events, however, since it excluded people who experienced only 'ambiguous' events. This potential problem is indicative of an approach based on researcher rather than on respondent assessments.

Another methodological problem in the Lambeth study involved the timing of the support measure in relation to the life event. This problem exists because the availability of support is not static and may be influenced by life events. Measuring support prior to the occurrence of life events which involve the loss of a close social tie, such as the death of a spouse, may thus overestimate the availability of support. On the other hand, the experience of life events may stimulate a person's network of relatives and friends, creating new forms of social participation and changing the quantity and quality of the individual's social ties. In the absence of precise information on the availability of social ties to buffer the experience of life events, the respondents' average support over the first and second interviews was employed. Such a broad measurement meant, however, that the changes in support categories between interviews were fairly small.

Analyses of changes in functioning among the life-event and no-life-event groups showed that the life-event group experienced a greater decline in functioning. The difference was, however, statistically significant only for changes in psychosocial functioning. A high level of social contact among this group was significantly related to a smaller decline in psychosocial functioning, after controlling for age, sex, and initial level of disability. This pattern was also true for physical functioning, but the difference was not statistically significant. As Table 9.2 shows, a high level of support was also associated with a smaller decline in functioning among no-life-event respondents, although the differences between support groups were not statistically significant. These results suggest that social contact is protective regardless of life events, but has its greatest effect on the psychosocial functioning of respondents who have recently experienced an adverse life event. Similar analyses using a measure of emotional support, based on the availability of people to confide in, showed a similar pattern, although the differences were not statistically significant (Patrick *et al.* 1984).

To determine the existence of a possible confounding effect between the measure of support and health outcomes, the analysis was repeated using the respondent's emotional functioning score as the dependent variable, which was a sub-category of the global psychosocial score that contained items relating only to emotion and alertness. The findings for emotional functioning closely followed those for the global measure of psychosocial functioning. Thus the greatest decline in functioning occurred among people who experienced an adverse life event but had a low level of social contact (Table 9.2).

Table 9.2. *Mean changes in health status scores between first and second interviews by level of support and presence of adverse life event (controlling for age, sex, and initial level of disability)*

	Average level of social contact at 1st and 2nd interview (1)	Physical score	Psychosocial score	Emotional score
		(larger values indicate decreased functioning)		
Adverse Life event	High (N = 24)	3.62	3.02	5.49
	Low (N = 40)	4.90	13.47*	16.40*
No adverse life event	High (N = 234)	2.05	4.50	5.31
	Low (N = 285)	3.17	6.84	7.51

* $p < .01$ comparing high and low levels of social contact among group experiencing an adverse life event.
(1) High support defined as a score over 30 on the five-item social contact measure and low support as a score of 0–30 (see Fig. 9.1).

Analyses of the relationship between support and changes in functioning among disabled people in the Lambeth study thus provides evidence of a small, but positive, relationship between level of social contact and changes in physical and psychosocial functioning. Examination of the interaction between support, life events, and changes in health status, however, showed that the strongest and only significant association was the positive effect of a high level of social contact on psychosocial and emotional functioning among people who had experienced a life event. Although this indicates that the major impact of support over a short time period is to moderate the adverse effects of life crises on individual functioning, support may also have a long-term cumulative and protective effect which is independent of life events. This long-term, independent effect of support may be particularly important among disabled people who by definition experience restrictions in functioning, and may need to adjust to a new more limited social role and to a variety of uncertainties and fears. However, although the relative importance of the buffering and direct effects of support appears to be influenced by the study design and measures employed, it is now well established that support can have a protective effect on health, and especially on psychiatric states and feelings of well-being.

Nature and dynamics of support

Relatively little attention has been paid to the process by which support exerts a protective effect, although the concept of coping is often invoked as the effective mechanism. Coping is defined by Lazarus (1981) as 'efforts, both action-oriented and intrapsychic, to manage environmental and internal demands and conflicts among them, which tax or exceed a person's resources'. Such coping may be adaptive, involving positive responses to changed circumstances and attitudes and behaviours that promote normal functioning. However, coping may also be maladaptive, giving rise to feelings of worthlessness, psychological distress, and excessive dependence.

Social ties may promote adaptive coping behaviour at a psychological level by strengthening the individual's internal resources. For example, such ties may improve the individual's self-concept, which may be viewed as originating from and sustained in social interaction. Social ties or the feeling and integration they provide may also give the individual a sense of certainty and purpose in living. The protective effects of the individual's psychological well-being, in terms of promoting morale, self-esteem, and feelings that life is meaningful, have been demonstrated by studies examining the effects of patients' psychosocial state on recovery from surgery and heart attacks (Mumford *et al.* 1982; Hyman 1975).

Psychological support may also promote coping by reducing the perceived threat of the problem or loss. This process occurs through talking with others, which helps to ease situations, making adverse events appear less unacceptable and more understandable. An example is 'grief work', which allows bereaved people to work through their grief, accept their loss, and look towards new goals (Gerhardt 1979). In the case of serious illness and disability, such support may also assist positive adjustment, which often requires the acceptance of a new self-image and lifestyle, and the reassurance that they continue to be valued and of importance to others.

At a social level, coping resources provided by social ties consist of instrumental support and problem solving, which are both designed to change the situation rather than its meaning. For example, after initially adjusting to a loss or a severe decline in functioning, people often must reorganize their lives, which includes adopting new roles and activities. They may require assistance with practical tasks, with gaining entry into new social groups, and with establishing a new pattern of life. Social ties may aid in these tasks directly, as well as providing advice and links to formal organizations and professional groups.

The need for social or psychological resources, or some combination of the two, to help people cope depends on the nature of the problem and the stage they have reached in coping with it. For example, a few strong supportive ties may be particularly important when a person feels an overriding need for emotional assurance, such as during the early stages of widowhood or unemployment, during the initial adjustment to surgical procedures, or when faced with physical impairments that affect the individual's self-image. At later stages, however, the existence of a larger, more diverse network may be important, for it is likely to encompass many different skills and sources of helpful advice. As Walker, *et al.* (1977) comment, in regard to the later stages of widowhood, a 'small dense network may entrap the individual within a limited set of normative expectations, information and social contacts, rather than fulfil his need to make a transition to new social roles'.

Epidemiological studies have emphasized the positive rather than adverse effects of social ties on health and well-being. However, social ties may contribute directly to the onset of illness by creating additional stress and tensions, while many life events are themselves associated with changes in social relationships (e.g., marital breakdown and death of spouse). Social ties may also encourage unfavourable coping responses that adversely affect the recovery or functioning of disabled people. Studies of hospital patients have shown that positive family attitudes are associated with good outcomes, while negative or overly protective attitudes are associated with poor outcomes (New *et al.* 1968). Overly protective attitudes towards disabled people may inhibit their attempts to achieve normal functioning. Likewise, unrealistic expectations may produce a sense of failure and inhibit positive coping efforts.

The proposition that social ties exert a protective effect on health thus need qualifying, for it is important that the support is appropriate to the individual's needs and promotes positive coping. It is therefore necessary to determine more precisely how and to what extent different forms of support promote health and feelings of well-being during different stages of illness. For example, strong psychological support from a few close relatives may be particularly important for people with severely disabling conditions or at the onset of disability. Social participation, practical advice, and assistance in attaining new goals may be of greater importance, however, for those who are mildly disabled. Other questions concern the interaction between the individual's social circumstances and economic resources, and the social and psychological support provided by social ties. In some cases, inadequate coping behaviour may not reflect the lack or inappropriateness of support as much as the restricted opportunities and problems arising from the individual's social position. Coping efforts may be restricted, for example, by financial or transportation problems, or by a lack of job opportunities or problem-solving skills.

Social ties among disabled people

Despite the importance of social ties to disabled people, little is known about the nature of their networks and sources of psychological and social support. In particular, we need to ask whether increasing disability is associated with changes in levels of support, whether the lack of different forms of support is concentrated among particular groups, and what characterizes people with low levels of support.

The social ties of disabled people, like other groups, are

influenced by general social processes, including changes in family size, the extent of geographical mobility, housing policies, and the existence of community groups and organizations. In the Borough of Lambeth, for example, two characteristics likely to influence social network patterns are the re-housing programmes of the early 1960s, which broke up many traditional communities, and the ethnic diversity of the population. Altogether, 8 per cent of the disabled respondents in the Lambeth survey, aged 45–75, were born in the West-Indies, and 3 per cent in India, Pakistan, or Bangladesh. The various ethnic minorities are concentrated in distinct areas of Lambeth. They exhibit different cultural patterns, although they share some experiences associated with their recent immigration and minority status.

The support available to different groups in Lambeth was examined using four measures, each reflecting a different concept of support (Fig 9.1). Information on social contact and the numbers of people in whom the respondent would confide was collected at all three phases of the study. Questions about feelings of loneliness were asked at the second phase and about the respondents' main confiding relationship at the third phase.

The distribution of scores revealed that disabled people of foreign birth felt they had a greater number of people to confide in than did their British-born counterparts. This reflected the close kin ties among the former group, with 26 per cent having three or more kin living in the same or an adjacent borough compared with only 15 per cent of the British-born respondents. Foreign-born respondents, however, had a slightly lower social contact score than the British born, associated with their lower employment rate and more limited participation in activities outside the home.

Table 9.3 shows the support available to people with different levels of physical functioning. As expected, people with minimal restrictions had a higher level of social contact than people with more severe disability. This was mainly due to the higher employment rate among the least disabled people, with 38 per cent of people with a physical score of under 20 working full- or part-time compared with only 8 per cent of those with a score of 35 and over (Table 9.4). There was little difference between network emotional support scores or in the availability and strength of the main confiding relationship for people with different levels of physical functioning. People with minimal physical restrictions

Table 9.3. *Support scores by level of physical functioning among respondents age 45–75 in Lambeth Health Survey*

| Support scores (1) | Physical score | | | |
	Under 20	20–34	35 and over	All levels
	Second interview			
	(N = 364)	(N = 112)	(N = 82)	(N = 55)
Social contact score	%	%	%	%
0–30 (low)	47	68	70	55
30–45	27	24	24	26
over 45	25	8	6	19
Network emotional support score				
0–4 (low)	62	68	70	64
5–9	35	29	25	32
10 or more	4	4	5	4
Loneliness				
Much/a lot of time	24	41	30	28
Some/little of time	11	13	23	13
Never lonely	65	46	46	58
	Third interview			
	(N = 292)	(N = 109)	(N = 93)	(N = 49)
Main confiding relationship	%	%	%	%
0 (no main confidant)	9	14	6	9
1–5 (satisfies some dimensions)	36	33	38	30
6 (satisfies all dimensions)	64	53	55	60

(1) See Fig. 9.1. for description of measures of support.

were, however, less likely to feel lonely, which was associated with their higher level of social contact and participation in employment.

Marital state formed the most important socio–demographic characteristic associated with differences in network size and

Table 9.4. *Sources of social contact by level physical functioning among respondents aged 45–75 in Lambeth Health Survey (second interview)*

Sources of social contact	Physical score			
	Under 20	20–34	35 & over	All levels
	(N = 364)	(N = 112)	(N = 82)	(N = 55)
Household size	%	%	%	%
1	27	28	29	28
2	40	41	41	40
3	17	14	12	16
4 or more	26	17	18	25
Network members outside household seen last week				
0	3	3	2	3
1–3	37	36	42	37
4–6	38	40	39	38
7 or more	22	21	17	21
Employment				
Not working	61	94	92	72
Part-time work	7	1	2	5
Full-time work (30 hours or more)	32	5	6	23
Attendance at religious service/activities+				
Less than once a year	62	71	70	65
At least once a year	15	12	7	13
At least once a month	23	17	23	22
Use of social services in last 14 days+				
District nurse	1	3	10	3
Home help	5	17	26	10
Meals on wheels	–	6	16	4
Luncheon club/ Day centre	6	3	7	17

+ Categories are not mutually exclusive

support among disabled respondents, as among the population as a whole (Morgan, 1980; Morgan *et al.* 1984). At each level of physical functioning married people tended to have larger networks than the non-married (single, widowed, and divorced) and relied more on kin for support. Non-married people living alone had the smallest networks and lowest levels of social contact and emotional support. They were also more likely to identify friends rather than kin as sources of support. These differences in the availability of support between household groups held for two broad age groups (45–64 and 65–74) and for the main ethnic groups.

Married people were least likely to feel lonely. However, there was little difference in feelings of loneliness between non-married people who lived with others and those who lived alone, despite the higher level of support reported by those sharing a household with others (Table 9.5). This draws attention to an important distinction between the number and type of social ties a person may have and their subjective feelings of being alone or lonely, which is often associated with the loss of close ties. It also shows that people's perceived needs for social ties may vary considerably according to their general life experiences, health, and other circumstances.

Information on social ties thus indicates that non-married people living alone have the smallest networks and are most likely to have a low level of support. There was, however, little difference in the number of close ties and support available to people with different levels of physical functioning, apart from differences arising from employment. The absence of marked differences in other sources of support may reflect two forces. On the one hand, a number of processes may reduce the social ties and support available to severely disabled people. These include physical restrictions (such as difficulty walking, blindness, and giddiness) that limit participation in work and social activities outside the home. In addition, disabling conditions that interfere with normal social interaction, such as deafness and blindness, or that are associated with considerable pain or emotional disturbance, are likely to inhibit an individual's ability or even desire to create and maintain large numbers of social ties. In the Lambeth survey, for example, 31 per cent of the disabled respondents, aged 45–74, interviewed at the second phase of the study said they were

Table 9.5. *Support scores for household groups among disabled people aged 45–75 in Lambeth Health Survey*

Support scores	Married	Household group Non-married lives with others	Non-married lives alone
	Second interview (N = 301)	(N = 108)	(N = 150)
Social contact score	%	%	%
0–30 (low)	40	42	93
30–45	32	38	6
over 45	28	20	1
Network emotional support score			
0–4 (low)	55	61	86
5–9	40	33	13
10 or more	5	6	1
Loneliness			
Much/a lot of time	22	40	31
Some/little of time	7	17	22
Never lonely	70	43	47
	Third interview (N = 256)	(N = 105)	(N = 150)
Main confiding relationship	%	%	%
0 (no main confidant)	3	9	21
1–5 (satisfies some dimensions)	22	33	40
6 (satisfies all dimensions)	75	58	39

taking part in fewer community activities because of their health, and 40 per cent were visiting people outside the home less often.

Whereas some processes reduce the number and quality of social ties among disabled people, others increase them. For example, a chronic illness may lead to a greater closeness with family members and a strengthening of social bonds. The apparent effects of disability on social ties may also be camouflaged by the fact that people with few social ties are less likely to be included in a community sample due to their higher rates of mortality and institutional admission. The outcome of these different processes results in a fairly wide distribution of support scores, with even some married and minimally disabled people exhibiting low levels of support, while some severely disabled people reported high levels of support. Furthermore, in some cases people possessed a high level of one form of support but not of another. For example, 31 per cent of respondents with a network of emotional support score of 5 or more did not have a single, strong, confiding relationship (score of 6), and conversely 12 per cent of those with a strong confiding relationship had a network emotional score of less than 5 (Morgan *et al.* 1984). This draws attention to differences between the quantity and quality of supportive ties and indicates there is no simple answer to the question of who lacks support. Furthermore, various groups are likely to have different needs for support. For example, some may desire to be part of a large social network, whereas other may not wish to fulfil the reciprocal obligations such membership implies. A life-long pattern of social isolation is also quite different from recent involuntary reductions in social interaction. Individual perceptions and satisfaction with support are thus likely to reflect their particular circumstances and experiences, and to vary according to their life-cycle stage and health state. A greater understanding of these issues, however, must await more detailed studies.

Promoting social ties

Methods of increasing or strengthening people's social ties may take a number of forms depending on each person's situation and needs. One approach is to encourage and aid the participation of disabled people in activities outside the home through reducing social, economic, and physical barriers. This strategy may involve providing transportation and taking other measures to increase disabled people's mobility and access, devising schemes to increase employment opportunities, and aiding their participation in social groups and organizations, so as to increase their integration into the wider society. Such measures have received greater emphasis in Britain since the early 1970s than before, as evidenced by regulations governing the construction of public buildings, by the increasing number of holiday and social club schemes for disabled people, and by attempts to educate the public so as to reduce the stigma attached to disabling conditions.

A second approach is to promote particular types of social ties. This may involve establishing home visiting schemes for the housebound, or counselling and assistance for those going through a period of crisis. Of particular importance in recent years has been the marked expansion of self-help groups, many of which cater for people with particular types of chronic conditions (e.g., multiple sclerosis, stroke victims, diabetes) or common life situations (e.g., widows, families with a handicapped child). These groups are based on the principle of mutual aid, where the helper is also one of the helped, with the emphasis being on providing practical assistance, advice, and emotional support to members. In one of the few controlled trials of a self-help intervention programme for widows, Vachon *et al.* (1980) found that widows assigned to an experimental widow-to-widow program adapted in ways similar to control subjects who had received no intervention. However, the rate of achieving landmark stages was accelerated for the intervention group, which suggests that such programmes may play an important role in improving health, coping ability, and life in general for disabled people. Although focussing on mutual aid, most self-help groups are also involved to some extent in political and educational activities to improve the lives of their members by lobbying for better provisions and reducing the disadvantages and handicaps experienced (McEwan *et al.* 1983).

A third approach is to strengthen existing social ties. Health professionals can influence the nature and quality of informal support, for example, by giving information and advice to the relatives of disabled people and ensuring that the relatives have realistic expectations of the disabled person's level of functioning and needs. For families caring for a severely dependent relative, family support can also be strengthened by reducing the family's burden of care. For instance, short-term residential or 'respite' care could be obtained for dependent people during holidays to relieve the family periodically. However, while such measures alleviate the burden of care, they do not change the fundamental problems experienced in the long-term care of severely disabled people.

Whatever approach is adopted, it is essential for the programmes to match people's perceived needs, desire for support, and health conditions. In addition, an emphasis on interventionist measures to strengthen and increase people's social ties must not detract attention from the wider social processes that produce social isolation and loneliness among large sections of the population. These include geographical mobility and rehousing programmes, fear of violence on the streets, general social attitudes towards the aged, and a lack of a 'sense of community', which is prevalent in many urban areas. Furthermore, effective coping often depends not only on the support provided by close social ties, but also on the individual's economic resources, housing conditions, and employment opportunities. Social ties and the support they provide thus can be viewed as one element in a complex armoury of resources that promote feelings of well-being and enable people to cope with chronic illness and life crises.

References

Andrews, G., Tennant, C., Hewson, D., and Vaillant, G., (1978). Life-event stress, social support, coping style, and risk of psychological impairment. *The Journal of Nervous and Mental Disease* **166**, 307–16.

Berkman, L. K. and Syme, L. (1979). Social networks, host resistance, and mortality: a nine-year follow-up study of Alameda County residents. *American Journal of Epidemiology* **109**, 186–204.

Brown, G. W. and Harris, T. (1978). *The social origins of depression.* Tavistock, London.

Cohen, S. and Syme, S. L. (eds) (1985). *Social support and health.* Academic Press Inc., London.

Durkheim, E. (1897, trans. 1951). *Suicide.* The Free Academic Press Inc., New York.

Faris, R. and Dunham, H. (1939). *Mental disorders in urban areas.* University of Chicago Press, Chicago.

Gehardt, U. (1979). Coping and social action: theoretical reconstruction of the life-event approach. *Sociology of Health and Illness* **i**, 195–225.

Goldberg, E. and Comstock, G. V. (1980). Epidemiology of life events: frequency in general populations. *American Journal of Epidemiology* **3**, 736–52.

Gore, S. (1978). The effects of support in moderating the health consequences of unemployment. *Journal of Health and Social Behaviour* **19**, 157–65.

Harris, A. (1971). *Handicapped and impaired in Great Britain.* HMSO, London.

Holohan, C. and Moos, R. (1981). Social support and health. *Medical Care* 15, (suppl), 47–58.

Holmes, T. and Rahe, R. (1967). The social readjustment rating scale. *Journal of Psychosomatic Research* 11, 3–218.

Hyman, M. (1975). Social psychological factors affecting disability among ambulatory patients. *Journal of Chronic Disease* 28, 213–8.

Kaplan, H., Cassel, J., and Gore, S. (1977). Social support and health. *Medical Care* 15, (suppl), 47–58.

Kasl, S. (1982). Social and psychological factors affecting the course of disease: an epidemiological perspective. In *The handbook of health care and the health profession.* (ed. D. Mechanic). Free Press, Riverside, New Jersey.

La Rocco, J., House, J., and French, J. R. (1980) Social support, occupational stress, and health. *Journal of Health and Social Behaviour* 22, 202–18.

Lazarus, R. S. (1981). The stress and coping paradigm. In *Theoretical bases for psychopathology* (eds. C. Eisdorfer, D. Cohen, A. Kleinman, and P. Maxim). Spectrum, New York.

Linn, N., Simeone, R., Emel, W., and Kuo, W. (1979) Social support, stressful life events, and illness: a model and an empirical test. *Journal of Health and Social Behaviour* 20, 108–19.

McEwen, J., Martini, C., and Williams, N. (1983). *Participation in health.* Croom Helm, London.

Morgan, M. (1980). Marital status, health, illness and service use. *Social Science and Medicine* 14A, 633–43.

Morgan, M., Patrick, D. L., and Charlton, J. (1984). Social networks and psychosocial support among disabled people. *Social Science and Medicine* 19, 489–97.

Mumford, E., Schlesinger, S., and Glass, G. (1982). The effects of psychological intervention on recovery from surgery and heart attacks: an analysis of the literature. *American Journal of Public Health* 72, 141–51.

Najman, J. M. (1980). Theories of disease causation and the concept of general susceptibility. *Social Science and Medicine* 14A, 231–7.

New, P., Ruscio, R., Prest, R., Petrisi, D., and George, L. (1968). The support structure of heart and stroke patients. *Social Medicine* 2, 185–200.

Nissel, M. and Bonnerjea, L. (1982). *Family care of the handicapped elderly: who pays?* Policy Studies Institute, London.

Nuckolls, L., Cassel, J., and Kaplan, B. H. (1971). Psychosocial assets, life crises and pregnancy. *American Journal of Epidemiology* 95, 431–41.

Patrick, D. L., Morgan, M., and Charlton, J. R. (1986). Psychosocial support and change in the health status of physically disabled people. *Social Science and Medicine* **22**, 1347–54.

Thoits, P. (1982) Conceptual, methodological and theoretical problems in studying social support as a buffer against life stress. *Journal of Health and Social Behaviour* **23**, 145–59.

Vachon, M., Lyall, W., Rodgers, J., Freedman-Letofsky, K., and Freeman, S. (1980). A controlled study of self-help for widows. *American Journal of Psychiatry* **137**, 1380–4.

Walker, A. (1987) Enlarging the Caring Capacity of the Community: Informal support networks and the welfare state. *International Journal of Health Services* 17, 369–87.

Walker, K., MacBride, A., and Vachon, M. (1977). Social support and the crisis of bereavement. *Social Science and Medicine* **11**, 35–42.

Williams, A., Ware, J. E., and Donald, C. A. (1981). A model of mental health, life events, and social supports applicable to general populations. *Journal of Health and Social Behaviour* **22**, 324–36.

10

Coping with Disability and Handicap

DAVID LOCKER

This chapter examines the nature and determinants of handicap. In particular, it explores the problems that chronically sick and disabled people encounter in everyday life, the resources which compensate for their functional losses, and their efforts to cope with those losses. The information is based on a series of semi-structured interviews with 16 women and 8 men who were moderately to severely disabled by rheumatoid arthritis. The main aim of the interviews was to explore the meaning of chronic illness and disability by documenting the impact of rheumatoid arthritis on everyday life and life prospects. (For a fuller account of the study and data, see Locker 1983.)

We decided to study people with rheumatoid arthritis because of the disease's various debilitating characteristics. Rheumatoid arthritis produces inflammation and swelling in the supporting tissues of the joints throughout the body. Its main symptoms are unremitting pain, stiffness and deformity of joints, loss of strength, dexterity, and mobility, and a loss of energy due to the metabolic effects of the disorder. A relatively common disease that can be severely disabling at an early age, it is a progressive, fluctuating condition with an unknown aetiology. The only available treatments are palliative and often unsuccessful. Furthermore, the disease can cause visible deformities. Given the aim of the study, individuals were selected who had been appreciably disabled by the disease for a number of years. They were identified via the screening study described in Chapter 2, by the caseloads of the rehabilitation officers employed by the Social Services Department, and by the local branch of the British Rheumatism and Arthritis Association. The onset of significant disability varied from 2 to 30 years when the study began.

While 7 of the people contacted were able to walk outside the house unaided, 4 were confined to wheelchairs, and the remainder did not or could not go outside without help. At times, all of them experienced difficulty moving around indoors. Twelve people were married, 6 single, 4 widowed, and 2 divorced. Nine lived alone, and the remainder lived with one or more relatives. Eleven were working-class, 13 middle-class, and only 1 was employed full-time. Each person was interviewed in his or her home immediately after the initial contact and again a year later. All interviews were tape-recorded and transcribed.

The International Classification of Impairments, Disabilities, and Handicaps, defines 'handicap' as the disadvantage experienced by impaired and disabled people because they do not or cannot conform to the expectations of the society or social groups to which they belong. Rheumatoid arthritis produces functional limitations in the trunk and limbs and eventually leads to restrictions in carrying out daily activities. The loss of mobility, ambulation, and manual dexterity, accompanied by weakness, is handicapping because it leads to social, psychological, and economic problems. People suffering from the disease may become unemployed or unable to follow the career of their choice. Thus, they may experience a substantial reduction in income and have only limited access to activities and facilities in the community. They may become socially isolated or dependent upon others, have low self-esteem, and experience significant changes in family relationships and social roles.

Empirical evidence of such deprivation abounds, and there can be no doubt that disabled people are a disadvantaged minority within British society. Studies by Sainsbury (1970), Harris (1971), and Townsend (1979) have demonstrated that in terms of income, employment, housing, and social and leisure opportunities, disabled people are markedly worse off than their non-disabled counterparts. Disabled people may also be forced to depend upon a system of welfare provision that perpetuates and exacerbates their dependency (Walker, 1980; Shearer 1981). While such studies have been and are essential to the political process of securing additional resources for disabled people, they fail to explore the nature of handicap and, by focusing on outcomes, neglect the variable sequence of events linking physical loss and malfunction with social disadvantage. They offer valuable evidence of handicap, but provide only a partial understanding of its character and consequences.

Handicap is far more pervasive than is suggested by the available statistics on unemployment, poverty, and poor housing. As some studies of the families of disabled children have revealed, a significant aspect of being or caring for a chronically ill person is the 'daily grind' or never-ending and unrewarded hard work involved in coping on a daily basis. For non-disabled people, the activities of daily living are usually taken for granted. But disabled people have so much trouble performing daily tasks that scarce resources, such as time, energy, and money, are totally consumed by the sheer effort of managing the disease day-to-day.

The volume and nature of the problems that a chronically ill person encounters is influenced, of course, by the severity of the disorder, the related symptoms, and the type of disability. The impact that these problems have on everyday life and life prospects also varies according to the context in which they exist. The disadvantage or handicap arising out of a given impairment or disability is both historically and culturally variable so that a certain attribute or incapacity may be handicapping in one society or social group but not in another, or at one point in time but not at another (Hanks and Hanks 1948; Freidson 1965). Similarly, the impact of an impairment or disability is influenced by more immediate social and environmental contexts. For example, the loss of one finger is likely to have different consequences for a manual labourer than for a professional musician. Likewise, an inability to climb stairs will impose more severe limitations on someone living on the fifth floor of a block of flats without a lift than on someone living on the ground floor. The meaning of a given functional limitation or activity restriction will also be influenced by the person's resources and coping strategies.

Living with rheumatoid arthritis

The problems experienced by people with rheumatoid arthritis can be placed in three broad categories roughly compatible with impairment, disability, and handicap: problems that arise directly from the disorder, problems that arise because of an inability to perform some daily living activities, and problems associated with the social consequences of disability such as unemployment, poverty, and dependence upon others. Rheumatoid arthritis has a number of distressing symptoms that have a profound impact on the course of everyday life. Even before the disease has caused any significant disability, the person must come to terms with severe pain, stiffness, uncertainty, and a lack of energy. As a result, disadvantage can arise directly from impairment without necessarily involving disability as an intermediary.

Pain associated with rheumatoid arthritis fluctuates. Acute phases in which the pain is severe and unremitting are followed by relatively quiescent phases in which pain levels subside and mobility improves. During either phase, pain might vary from day-to-day, to such an extent that all the respondents characterized their life in terms of 'good days' and 'bad days'. While they might reorganize their lives in the attempt to reduce pain, they rarely could avoid pain altogether. As one woman commented, 'Everything you do means pain'.

Because of the way that rheumatoid arthritis damages the supporting structures of the joints, mobility causes pain, but immobility results in stiffness, often making subsequent movement difficult and more painful. After a night's sleep, for example, joints are very stiff and considerable effort is required to loosen them in the mornings. Therefore, many of the respondents attempted to alternate periods of rest and movement during the day. Whenever possible, they avoided sitting for longer than an hour and would periodically walk around the room.

At times, however, the pain was so severe that it was more disabling than the damage to the joints. Limbs capable of movement were rendered immobile by actual or anticipated pain. One women, interviewed during an acute attack, said, 'For me to lean across the table and pick that up, which is something people would do without thinking about it, causes me pain and takes a tremendous effort to do it. And I don't want to do it because nobody, if they've got pain, wants to make it worse'. Even so, some activities are unavoidable, especially for the person who lives alone and must cope with basic essentials like toileting and eating. Then it is necessary to rally psychological resources in order to rise above pain and force the body to perform. One such women, struggling alone in her flat in the face of a number of chronic conditions, said, 'At the moment, I'm doing practically nothing because I can't. I'm having literally to screw up courage in the morning to get up to go into the bathroom. Every time I want to do something, I have to steel myself first to do it'. When these resources were not forthcoming, the person gave up, abandoning even simple activities like turning on the television or making a cup of tea. One man often missed his hospital appointments because the psychological and physical effort of getting there was too much.

The symptoms of rheumatoid arthritis would be easier to manage if they were not surrounded by uncertainty. The symptoms and effects vary not only from day-to-day, but also during the course of the day, so that the location and severity of the pain might change unpredictably. A 'good day' in the morning could easily become a 'bad day' by the afternoon. This variability and unpredictability adds to the cognitive problem of making sense of the disorder and the practical problem of containing its symptoms within acceptable boundaries. The disease requires constant monitoring because levels of pain and disability are never known in advance. Certainly, the problematic character of the symptoms maximizes their disruptive effect on personal and social life.

Knowledge is a powerful resource, helping both the emotional adaptation to, and practical management of, chronic illness (Bury 1982). As expected, many of the respondents attempted to impose a degree of certainty on their daily existence by identifying events that preceded acute phases or particularly painful days. Armed with such knowledge, they could at least acquire a measure of control over the situation. Some believed that cold or damp weather was responsible for increases in pain and some attributed these increases to emotional or physical stress. However, most were mystified and confused when their theories were rendered invalid by a bad day for which there was no apparent reason. One man said, 'You can never pin it down to one thing'. And one women complained, 'I don't understand why the pain isn't constant'. Such confusion meant that strategies or arrangements to control or accommodate to levels of pain were difficult to construct. Nevertheless, day-to-day experience was continually monitored and professional advice sought in the hope that a causal explanation would be forthcoming.

The majority of the people interviewed had been told by their doctors that rest was essential because excessive activity would inflame the joints and add to their disability. Many agreed with this advice and often found that activity on one day produced pain the next. Compliance with the advice was another matter, however, since inactivity meant boredom, frustration, and withdrawal from everyday life. As Weiner (1975) has described, people with rheumatoid arthritis must balance the physiological imperative and the activity imperative to maximize activity within an acceptable level of pain. Consequently, some followed their doctor's advice only selectively, saying 'I know this will have this effect on me, but I'll do it anyway'. The respondent who was employed full-time so disliked having to withdraw from family life on weekends in order to rest that she took one day of annual leave per week to stay at home. Consequently, she never had an extended holiday, but the strategy helped to keep her arthritis under control.

The variability and unpredictability of rheumatoid arthritis disrupted social life even more than the need to rest. Activities possible one day were impossible the next or impossible for 2 days running, but for different reasons. Shaving could be difficult one day because of a stiff shoulder and difficult another because painful fingers could not get a grip on a razor. To accommodate these shifting eventualities, the respondents had to redesign their coping strategies constantly. Some refused to plan ahead, living from day-to-day and doing what they could when they could. As one man said, 'Until you wake up in the morning, you don't know what you're going to wake up to. You couldn't say to someone, "Don't come tomorrow. I'm going to be bad" '. Some had an understanding with others whereby any arrangements made were subject to cancellation at short notice, and without causing offense they were able to ask family and friends not to visit. When one women found she could no longer safely make holiday plans in advance, the entire family pooled their resources and bought a caravan. The caravan was kept on the coast, available for her to use whenever she felt well.

One problem common to many disabled people is that of constructing a satisfactory life within the constraints of radically reduced physical resources. They must frequently allocate time or energy to some tasks at the expense of others. Fagerhaugh (1973) has described the way emphysema sufferers must select how they will use a limited oxygen supply, postponing other activities until their resources are replenished. The same process was observed among these rheumatoid arthritis sufferers. While they often ignored pain in order to accomplish necessary or valued activities, they could only do so much before the pain became too great. The day's quota of activity must be allocated to a few tasks, with the remainder left for another day. One woman allowed herself one walk per day, usually to do her shopping, after which she would need to rest for 2 hours for the pain to subside. On the day of the first interview, she had an appointment with an optician and the walk had to be reserved to get there. A desire to retain the integrity of the joints led some individuals to abandon some activities altogether. The respondent who worked full-time no longer made her dresses or knitted. 'I'd rather keep my hands for when I work', she said. Like the majority, she was a prisoner of time. Ordinary tasks took longer than normal to complete so that disproportionate amounts of time had to be set aside for mundane tasks such as washing and dressing. She always got up at 6.30 a.m., and she had to stick to a strict routine to be in the office by 9 o'clock. If she got up even 10 minutes late, she could not make up lost time by hurrying.

Acute attacks imposed even more constraints and made the choices even more stark. Constant pain depleted already diminished reserves of energy, and many preferred to be alone while in pain. One 53-year-old woman, confined to a wheelchair at the first interview and essentially bed-bound by the second, chose to spend most of the day in bed. She saved her energy for when her husband was at home in the evening.

People with rheumatoid arthritis also have to cope with the emotional problems created by a painful and disabling condition for which there is no cure. Weiner (1975) has shown how people with rheumatoid arthritis manage a problematic and uncertain future by social–psychological strategies designed to maintain hope. At the same time, they need strategies to manage a problematic present, allowing them to cope with chronic illness and disability while not being overwhelmed by the disease and its limitations. Many people learn to accept and live with rheumatoid arthritis by changing personal values and expectations in accordance with reduced abilities and become content to operate within new and narrowed boundaries of activity. For example, one basically house-bound woman was able to obtain pleasure and satisfaction by driving her daughter to the local shop. While accepting and living with arthritis, many respondents found it necessary to 'keep going' in spite of the pain and effort. They told stories of people who had 'given in', retired to bed, and become totally dependent upon others. The strategy of 'keeping going' is distinct from that described by Weiner (1975) as 'keeping-up'. The former is not an attempt to maintain normal levels of activity to conceal the disease from others, but rather an attempt to prevent stagnation, further loss of faculty, and the decline into the static existence of an invalid. A 39-year-old woman who insisted on doing her own housework, despite having five children aged 14 to 21 at home, expressed it this way:

'I scrubbed my kitchen on my hands and knees Thursday. It crippled me, but that's beside the point. I shall still do it because, if I don't do it, it's one more thing I can't do. If I didn't, I feel that eventually I shall finish up getting out of bed, walking downstairs, sitting there all day, and then at night walking back up again, and I'm not prepared to do that.'

Social resources and the practical problems of everyday life

Chronic illness leading to loss of physical capacity calls into question the personal, financial, and social resources of an individual. Resources that may have been adequate prior to onset are inadequate to compensate for physical loss and provide for a satisfactory existence in the community. The inadequacy of resources may become more acute over time as the increasingly disabled person sees the erosion of income, wealth, and, in some cases, social support. Thus, disabled people manage the illness and its effects with fewer resources than they enjoyed while they were able-bodied.

When people no longer have the strength or manual dexterity to perform everyday tasks or when they are immobilized by pain, the nature and extent of their resources will have a significant impact on the quality of everyday life. While there were wide variations in the resources available to individual respondents, few were content with what they had. Many were involved in a long and arduous struggle to obtain more appropriate housing, aids and appliances, additional financial benefits or allowances, and domiciliary services. For some, dealing with the complexities of the welfare bureaucracy and trying to get it to respond adequately to their needs absorbed a great deal of time and energy. As one man said, 'When you're ill, you get sick of the argy-bargy. And for everything, you've got to send them letters. You just keep sending letters *all* the time'.

Money and appropriate physical environments are key resources for people with chronic illness and disability because they aid independent living. Other key resources are personal help and social support. Those who lived with others or could call on spouses and/or children were more able to manage the practicalities of everyday life with minimum effort. For those who lived alone without sources of help, even the simplest task could present a major problem. Until he acquired the appropriate aids and appliances, one single man had to go through an hour of painful rolling and heaving just to get out of bed. One elderly widow who lost her only source of support when her husband died, described dressing and undressing as a 'nightmare'. It was impossible for her to get her stockings on and off without the help of the nurse who came to give her a weekly bath. Once on, she had to keep the stockings on for a week.

Nearly all of the respondents who lived alone and some of them who lived with others managed a household by lowering their standards of cleanliness and order, thereby reducing the need to expend valuable energy on housework. Conflicts with home-helps and family over how and when to do the cleaning and laundry diminished as this kind of work became unimportant. This shift in values caused difficulty for some of the housewives because it meant abandoning a highly valued role. For more essential activities such as shopping and food preparation, there was often no alternative but to elicit the help of others. Some kinds of forward planning were essential for disabled people who lived alone. One such woman was able to get to the local shops by following a planned route and resting along the way on low walls. She would buy a few items over and above her immediate needs to make sure her cupboards were well stocked. She would draw on these reserves when she was unable to get out of the house due to the weather or her pain. Even people who had assistance with shopping had to plan ahead. Goods that run out or had been forgotten could not be replaced on weekends or public holidays, and there was a limit to how far in advance meals could be prepared even if a refrigerator was available for storage. Sometimes, planning ahead was difficult because disability pensions or other financial benefits did not arrive when they were needed. On the days that the home-help came, for instance, the disabled respondents might not have enough money to allow the help to buy in bulk, in which case they might have to rely on neighbours to do the odd bit of shopping.

While most of the respondents who received help did so from spouses and daughters, many existed within more extensive social networks. Their networks and the extent to which they received help varied widely (see Chapter 9). Irrespective of the amount of support given, some of these people derived a sense of comfort and security from knowing that they could draw on this resource in times of crisis. One severely disabled man, who relied heavily on his wife, was so well integrated into a family network that his wife's prolonged illness did not cause additional problems:

'We always see the family. They come round here or we go up there. There's always somebody in here. We're never on our own. They mix in. They don't look on her as an outcast because I can't do what they do. If ever there's anything we want—if we're in trouble—we ring up and they're over. You know, no bother like that. If anything goes wrong with the car, I ring the wife's brother up. So I've got no worries or anything like that. When my wife was ill, her mother came over and helped out, so I had no worry there. My daughter used to come. My son would come down. We've never had a problem because we've got a good family. They're always helpful.'

That case sharply contrasts with that of another couple who had no relatives and whose friendship network had collapsed as the husband became severely disabled. They lived in a block of flats constructed especially for people with severe disabilities and were largely confined to the block and its immediate environment. Some of the other residents were able to drive or had relatives who would lift them into cars and take them out. This couple had no car, and even if one had been available, the man was so badly affected that 'I would need a couple of strong lads to put me in and take me out. So one just has to live as we live, a very restricted life. If we had relatives, it would make all the difference'. Although he had a wheelchair, the couple were limited by the hilly terrain surrounding their home and his inability to use a toilet without his wife's help. Pushing him to the local shopping district involved a great deal of effort, and because their enquiries had not produced an aid or appliance to solve the problem, he had to be taken home if he needed to go to the lavatory.

One reason members of some social networks did not provide much practical help is that they were not asked to help. Some of the people interviewed felt it was inappropriate to seek help from people who had families and responsibilities of their own. One man and his wife had 12 brothers and sisters between them, and although they could have been helped in a number of ways, they continued to struggle alone. The wife was so afraid to leave her husband that she disliked going out even to shop. For a time, she arranged for the woman next door, who was expecting her first baby, to sit with her husband while she shopped for herself and her neighbour. The arrangement ended after the baby was born because, the woman said, 'I wouldn't ask her now. It wouldn't be fair to her. I mean, she's got a family of her own to bring up'. The wife's fears for her husband's safety, coupled with her reluctance to seek help, meant that she became as isolated and confined as her disabled spouse. If she wanted to be out of the house for any length of time, she had to keep the children home from school. The stigma of being dependent upon others was obviously relevant in this case. Said the woman:

'I mean, they [the family] feel sorry for us, but there's nothing they can do money-wise or anything. Well, I wouldn't ask. It's pride more than anything . . . I wouldn't ask his family for anything. I wouldn't. I don't like to have people think I'm down. I mean I know I'm down. I mean, as long as my rent's paid and my children are fed I don't care.'

The woman continued to conceal her family's decline into poverty as she struggled to maintain standards on an inadequate income.

Coping by withdrawal

Dependency is one change in social relationships that may arise as a result of chronic illness and disability. Another is emotional and physical withdrawal from immediate and wider networks of relatives and friends. In the study group, this withdrawal took a number of forms designed to solve a number of problems. Some legitimated the extent of their pain and suffering to sceptics by staying silent. Some withdrew into themselves when pain made it difficult to interact, but physical withdrawal was difficult. The woman who remained employed would often avoid conversation with others in the office because 'you don't feel like laughing and joking'. When in pain, most would separate themselves from family and friends until the pain had begun to subside. Often they did not have enough energy to maintain a normal front and take interest in others. Moreover, many did not bother to wash or dress on 'bad days', and did not want to be seen in that state by anyone other than their family. At times, some found it difficult to tolerate even close family. Because they were irritable and ill-tempered, they would minimize overt conflict by staying out of the way. One man said:

'Little things get on your nerves, things you wouldn't usually take notice of. You lose your temper. I'm not keen on people coming in. If the wife's relatives come, I sit for a while and make an excuse and go to bed. I can't explain it. I just know I'm going to end up in a temper. I prefer to get out of the way rather than cause an argument.'

Such a strategy contributed to the isolation of the disabled person and the eventual disintegration of social networks. The man quoted above said he had lost a number of friends because he was not always able to tolerate their presence or their anxiety to help.

Over time, families seemed to come to terms with the conflict that arose because of pain and developed ways of managing or neutralizing it. One woman described how her husband was able to distinguish a 'normal disagreement', which originated in a real difference of opinion, from her irritability when she was in pain. Although she was often unreasonable, he was able to cope with her distress:

'He will never take me up. Rather than do that, he will go out of the room. And when he comes back, I will start up again. But he will never pick up the gauntlet under those circumstances. What he does is give me enough time to vent my irritation and come over and put his arms around me. That normally finishes up with me having a bit of a grizzle and it's all right.'

Despite the fact that such irritability and intolerance were tied to pain, the respondents could not absolve themselves of responsibility for the strain it imposed on family relationships. They felt they ought to be more reasonable and more able to control their temper. This feeling heightened their guilt, for it was one more way in which their illness impinged on the quality of life of their close associates. As the woman above said of her husband, 'He deserves better'.

While withdrawal from family and friends was usually a consequence of pain, withdrawal from the wider world was largely a result of embarrassment and stigma (Cunningham 1977). When her pain was bad and mobility somewhat impaired, one woman chose to remain at home. 'You don't want to go hobbling down the road like an old lady', she said. 'You feel people are staring at you.' One man stopped going to his usual pubs and clubs because:

'I just don't feel like going where there are people. Possibly this is the reason I don't go to the pub. I can't pick up a pint glass; it's impossible without both of my hands . . . [People] think you're a wino or something. I used to go to this club, but I don't like going down now. They're all dancing, and you're hopping about with a stick, you feel a bit out of place.'

Withdrawal from the world and confinement within the home also arose as a result of inadequate personal and social resources. Again, a limited reserve of energy was a key factor. The sheer effort involved in getting washed, dressed, and ready to go out was enough to keep the person at home. Some felt that family members had enough to do managing the household and providing personal care, and they were unwilling to burden them by requests to go out. Those who lived alone without support had to abandon previously enjoyed social and recreational activities. One such man was able to go on an organized outing to the coast, 'but only because they collected me at the door'. A similarly situated woman could not take advantage of a similar trip organized by residents in her block of flats because she had no one to help her:

'I dare not go because it means getting on a coach. There're steps about a foot high and nobody to lift me in and nobody to lift me out. And even if I'm allowed to take the wheelchair, there are seven or eight steps up to the hotel where we have lunch. Then there's nobody to push me from there to the convenience or whatever. So I've decided not to go, which is a pity as it happens only once a year.'

Coping by withdrawal was also a strategy adopted by the relatives and friends of respondents. Some of the people interviewed were bitter and confused when their social networks crumbled after discovering that they could no longer easily participate in activities. The breakdown of such networks was also the result of mutual withdrawal from a problematic relationship. One family withdrew because it appeared unable to come to terms with its inability to help the disabled mother or do anything to reduce her pain and limited mobility. Because she sensed that her situation caused them pain and embarrassment, she stopped asking them to visit. Her helplessness and their helplessness were mutually distressing.

The significance of work

Becoming unemployed is a major transition point in the careers of disabled people, radically transforming the character of their everyday existence and bringing with it poverty and a host of other problems. Work is a resource, giving meaning and structure to the day and aiding the acquisition of other resources, predominately social contacts, self-esteem, and financial independence. All of the respondents had worked at some time in their lives, and all but two had given up employment because of rheumatoid arthritis. A quarter of those without jobs had been unemployed for 3 years or less, and some of the unhappiest people were among this group. They had not adjusted their aspirations and expectations to their new realities. They continued to hope that medical intervention would improve their physical status and restore their capacity to work.

The significance of work on everyday life was expressed well by a man who had been unemployed for a year when first seen. He had been an assistant manager with a local company until his increasing immobility forced him to quit. He wanted to return to work but was uncertain of his ability to manage full-time. 'I've got in my own mind to find out if I can go back to work or not', he said. 'So the only way is to go back and find out, and if I can't do it, then I've bloody well had it. I've got to go on a completely different track and have a different attitude toward life.' This man felt that little was being done to improve his clinical condition or to clarify the uncertainty regarding his return to work. If he could work, the structure of his life would remain largely intact; if not, his actions and attitudes had to be adjusted accordingly. Until the dilemma was resolved, there appeared little he could do to help himself and little point in pursuing new objectives.

Remaining in work following the onset of disability often depends upon the tolerance and flexibility of colleagues and superiors and the social and other resources deliberately or fortuitously placed at the person's disposal. The same job in the same organization might be manageable or impossible according to the responses of others. One woman who had been a senior secretary in a large organization found some working situations markedly easier than others. Working for one boss, she had been given an electric typewriter, had a clerical assistant who was a helpful 'motherly soul', and had three friends on the same corridor who looked in from time to time and saved her many trips to the photocopier or the postal room. When this boss retired, she worked for a very busy and ambitious man and, without the support she had received in her previous office, she could not keep up and asked to be transferred. After a number of similar experiences, she took a year's sick leave and was eventually retired by her employer. Many others told similar stories of how they had been able to remain at work only because colleagues and superiors had been understanding and flexible, taking over difficult tasks or allowing them to modify working hours or office routines.

Besides relying on others to help them perform a work-related task, disabled people can cope with the problematic aspects of employment by negotiating an occupational role more suited to their physical limitations. After initially relying on his colleagues, one man who co-owned a company that installed and serviced launderettes took over a set of essential, but less demanding, tasks. Although the company did business throughout the UK, he was allowed to handle the London end of the trade so as to reduce the necessity for him to travel. People who were unwilling to depend on the goodwill of others often preferred this strategy because they wished to conceal the illness or avoid being dependent. The one woman who remained employed full-time did clerical work in the Civil Service and successfully negotiated her way through a succession of jobs until she found one she could manage:

'I don't want to say at work, "Can you do this? Would you mind doing that?" because it looks as if you're being, you know . . . because I look fairly well, you see. I don't look ill, and people say well, "What's wrong?" if you keep asking. I've adjusted myself at home in the way I live, but at work I don't want people to be aware that I've got arthritis. I don't want them to look on me as a poor little invalid.'

When a job cannot be modified and the individual refuses to depend on others, becoming unemployed is the next alternative. One man who was one of several caretakers in a large complex of flats received considerable help from the others after he left the hospital. But he preferred to resign rather than depend on their help. Subsequently, his wife left work because his variable needs for care and attention made her an erratic worker. Together they chose to manage a family and household on a substantially reduced income rather than draw upon available resources and compromise their independence:

'When he was getting his off days, I sort of phoned up my governor and said, "I won't be in today. He's not well." And the next day he'd be a lot better, and I'd go into work. And then the next, I was off when he got bad. I was mucking him about, you know. He was very kind to me, but they can't go on forever doing it. You can't keep accepting his kindness all the time. I said, "You might as well get yourself another barmaid and cleaner." I didn't want to pack up work. I mean I'd go to work if I could. The guy said I could go back to work anytime I want, but I know it'll be just like before, being carried again. You can't have people carrying you all the time.'

All of the respondents who had become unemployed were devastated by job loss. In addition to a loss of income and unaccustomed poverty, they became bored and lonely and were frustrated by suddenly being confined to the house. Others were affected by a loss of identity, achievement, and involvement, formerly derived from being employed. Most felt peripheral to everyday life, mere observers of the activities of others. All faced the problem of what to do with their time. In this respect, a lack of work was felt most acutely by the single men who lived alone.

They seemed to have few ways to occupy their time and give meaning to the day.

The disabled women more often immersed themselves in family life, and those who lived with others also seemed to have wider networks of friends and family who helped fill surplus time. One woman had no relatives other than her husband and mother, but did have many friends from the local church. On giving up her job, she became more involved in church activities and her days were busy with telephone calls and people who visited in connection with this work.

Her case can be contrasted with that of one of the single men. After leaving his job as a lift attendant, he suddenly discovered what it meant to live alone. No longer able to occupy his time with small repair jobs around his flat, he became increasing bored and lonely. His doctor arranged for him to attend a local day centre, but pain and immobility sometimes kept him home for days at a time. 'I go nuts, I go really barmy', he said. 'I don't know what to do with myself. I want to do things, but I can't. All you've got is the TV. You try and sleep the time away.'

Similarly, single people and those living alone were more likely to live in poverty following unemployment. Wholly dependent upon state benefits, they had to manage a household alone and were unable to call on wider networks to help them cope on an inadequate income. While all attempted to manage on a limited income by cutting down on so-called luxuries, and eventually disposing of essential though expensive items like telephones and cars, respondents living alone had to adopt more drastic measures to avoid accumulating debt. One woman said she had to 'ease up on the groceries' to pay the bills.

Chronic illness and the quality of everyday life

In a sense, the problems that members of the study group encountered were never solved; they were merely transformed and exchanged for problems of a different order. Using a walking stick or other such aids may have assisted mobility, but only at a cost of feeling stigmatized. Similarly, calling on others for assistance may ease the practical problems of daily living, but only at the cost of feeling guilty or a burden. And a resort to welfare services may increase the person's dependency.

The resources that disabled people command reflect life prospects before and after the onset of illness and disability. Such resources figure significantly in the strategies used to cope with problems because coping mechanisms inevitably draw on knowledge, psychological capacities, personal help, or material effects like money, adapted environments, and aids and appliances. The interviewees with the more extensive and varied resources were more successful at managing problems and able to select from a range of available strategies, often avoiding the negative outcomes associated with some. As Bury (1982) and Gerhardt (1979) have suggested, the distribution of resources in society and the differential ability of individuals from different socio–economic groups to modify their social environment and respond satisfactorily to changing circumstances, means that some people are likely to be more disadvantaged than others by a long-term disabling illness.

In describing the effects of a chronic disabling disorder, we have attempted to convey the significance of the concept of handicap in understanding and alleviating the problems created by chronic illness. The concept of handicap is crucial for a number of reasons. First, the consequences of a long-term illness are often more distressing than the disease itself or the activity limitations it produces. In fact, the rationale for treating disease and limiting disability is to minimize their impact on the individual and society at large. Second, despite significant advances in medical knowledge, primary and secondary prevention are limited. Alleviating the broader personal and social difficulties associated with disability provides one avenue for improving patient welfare. Third, the kinds of disadvantages experienced by disabled people (unemployment, poverty, social isolation, and low self esteem) have been identified as precursors of ill health. A feedback mechanism may exist whereby such consequences, acting in a variety of ways, cause the physical and functional status of the person to deteriorate. In this way, enhancing welfare may maintain or improve levels of health.

While medical and rehabilitation services aim to limit disease and disability, social and community services are oriented towards the reduction of handicap. A number of organizations deal with the problems encountered by disabled people, and they are responsible for administering a complex and confusing system of social and economic provision. All the people interviewed drew to a greater or lesser extent on the services provided by central and local government. For some respondents, these were the only sources of financial and social support available. This group was more critical of the services they received than those who had somewhere else to turn.

Respondents suggested that the agents and agencies comprising the welfare bureaucracy created as many problems as they solved. While few identified gaps in services, all were critical of the way services were organized and delivered. To most, the system appeared to be unacceptable, inefficient, inflexible, and unresponsive to their needs. The whole process seemed to be governed by a set of rules and regulations that were irrational or arbitrary, and either prevented access to much needed resources or created unacceptable delays after eligibility for a service or a benefit was granted. Acquiring services and benefits often proved to be a long and exhausting process, and many complained of the stigma created when officials carelessly handed out moral judgments as well as financial and other support. Some respondents had the skills and social resources to manage the welfare bureaucracy and its agents and had become adept at getting the system to respond to their needs. Others simply withdrew and ceased to pursue their claims. They were left with a deep sense of injustice and felt abandoned by society and its caring institutions.

Clearly, money and social support are the two most significant resources for improving the lot of disabled people. The design and delivery of services to meet these needs involves a number of complex policy issues. Enough, however, has been written about the barriers to integration and the wider social origins of disadvantage to enable policy-makers to identify more effective policy options. Some people call for a shift of resources to make community care a reality, and some support a comprehensive disability income based on need, not on circumstances or place of onset. The challenge is not only to provide services that meet needs, but also to provide them in a manner that does not create dependency and a devalued status. We have long recognized that institutional care dehumanizes and depersonalizes by making the individual subordinate to a system that meets the needs of the organization, not the recipient. The same is true of community services, which also limit independence, constrain choice, and deprive the individual of dignity.

Because the volume and nature of welfare provision for people with disabilities is constrained, cost and social values are important factors to consider (Topliss 1985). We need to develop the ICIDH model and learn more about the dynamics of handicap even within the framework of a system of formal provision that is far from ideal. As Bury (1982) has suggested, we know little about the tolerance of families, friends, and colleagues and how they vary between social groups and settings. We know little about the development of social isolation, the fragmentation of networks following the onset of disability, or ways of helping individuals retain old or create new systems of social support. Berkman (1981; 1984), reviewing the literature linking health and social support, has shown that a variety of strategies may be necessary to modify the particular social or psychological processes at work in the individual case. By means of such strategies, individuals can be helped to maximize and mobilize key resources and to develop mechanisms to cope more effectively with the problematic aspects of everyday life. Accordingly, we need studies of disadvantage that use larger and randomly selected samples and that employ some measure of handicap. Such a measure would need to go beyond current indicators such as income, unemployment, and social isolation to encompass the more pervasive effects of chronic illness. In short, we need a technology to assign a numerical value to the meaning and consequences of disability that is sensitive to the context in which the disability occurs. This technology would apply equally to all the factors that intervene between impairment, disability, and handicap, be they social or psychological. Only then will it be possible to identify key variables and the part they play in the development of handicap, and only then will it be possible to create interventions to help disabled people limit the consequences of impairment and disability. In conjunction with services designed to promote independence, mobility, and opportunities for meaningful work, such an approach should help the integration of people with disabilities into the community and reduce their handicaps.

References

Berkman, L. (1981) Physical health and the social environment. In *The relevance of social science to medicine*. (eds L. Eisenberg and A. Kleinman) Reidel and Company, Dordrecht, Holland.

Berkman, L. (1984). Assessing the physical health effects of social networks and social support. *Annual Review of Public Health* **5**, 413–32.

Bury, M. (1982). Chronic illness as biographical disruption. *Sociology of Health and Illness* **4**, 167–82.

Cunningham, D. (1977). *Stigma and social isolation: self-perceived problems of a group of multiple sclerosis sufferers*. Health Services Research Unit, University of Kent, Canterbury.

Fagerhaugh, S. (1973). Getting around with emphysema. *American Journal of Nursing* **73**, 94–7.

Freidson, E. (1965). Disability as social deviance: In *Sociology and rehabilitation* (ed. M. Sussman). ASA, Washington.

Gerhardt, U. (1979). Coping as social action. *Sociology of Health Illness* **1**, 85–99.

Hanks, J. and Hanks, L. M. (1948). The physically handicapped in certain non-accidental societies. *Journal of Social Issues* **4**, 61–7.

Harris, A. (1971). *Handicapped and impaired in Great Britain. Part I*. HMSO, London.

Locker, D. (1983) *Disability and disadvantage: the consequences of chronic illness*. Tavistock Publications, London.

Sainsbury, S. (1970). *Registered as disabled*. Occasional papers in social administration. No. 35. G Bell and Sons, London.

Shearer, A. (1981) *Disability: whose handicap?* Basil Blackwell, Oxford.

Topliss, E. (1975). *Provision for the disabled*. Basil Blackwell and Martin Robertson, Oxford and London.

Townsend, P. (1979). *Poverty in the United Kingdom*. Allen Lane, London.

Walker, A. (1980) Social creation of poverty and dependency in old age. *Journal of Social Policy* **9**, 172–88.

Wiener, C. (1975). The burden of rheumatoid arthritis: tolerating the uncertainty. *Social Science and Medicine* **9**, 77–104.

11

A strategy for community provision

HEDLEY PEACH AND DONALD L. PATRICK

In our larger national life we will always remain largely
strangers to each other, and we will need a bureaucracy, with
all the impersonalness it implies, to mediate whatever
cohesiveness can be achieved by just policies of health care.
Nonetheless, such cohesiveness can be substantial, and
'community' is not too grandiose an idea—when shorn of its
utopian connotations—to express what is intended. A more
realistic sense of community is one in which there are shared
perceptions of the value of individual lives and a social
commitment to protect them all equitably. Equitable recognition of needs is a prerequisite for community and equitable
care for those needs is its goal.

Larry R. Churchill, *Rationing Health Care in America*

The way our culture gives definition to the process of growing 'old'
and being 'disabled' determines how stereotypes are formed for
elderly and disabled people. These stereotypes are shared by many
persons in the community, often by disabled people themselves. In
general, the experience of policy-makers, planners, and administrators who are concerned with elderly and disabled people has led
them to develop a pessimistic image of their clients. Professionals
in the health and social services, for example, work with elderly
and disabled people who are primarily ill or neglected, or whose
families cannot support them any longer. Similarly, policy-makers
and planners have gained much of their knowledge about elderly
and disabled people from research, most of which has been cross-
sectional studies of one sample of elderly or disabled people at one
point in time. Because of its policy focus on the 'need' for care,
this research has tended to concentrate on some of the most

vulnerable sub-groups, frequently clients of social services departments rather than elderly or disabled people in general. Few
studies track fluctuations in disability over time to observe the
appreciable proportion of disabled people who overcome many of
their functional limitations and activity restrictions. Without
longitudinal surveys and qualitative studies, the negative images
that policy-makers and planners have of elderly and disabled
people are reinforced. Their perceptions of the problems of
advancing age and of being disabled are often *too* pessimistic, just
as people whose elderly or disabled family members are competent
and happy may *minimize* the problems of elderly and disabled
people.

Neither an optimistic nor a pessimistic perception closely
approximates the truth, because neither encompasses the wide
variations that exist. Unfortunately, a generally negative image of
elderly and disabled people has become popular. The typical older
or disabled person in Britain is thought to suffer from poor health
and poor housing, to live alone on an inadequate income, to be
lonely and socially isolated, and to be a burden. But a growing
body of reseach on aging is leading to a reassessment of the
stereotypes of elderly people. The Lambeth studies of disablement
continue this reassessment with a focus on disabled adults in
general, a group defined by impairment, disability, and handicap
rather than by age.

In the International Classification of Impairments, Disabilities,
and Handicaps (ICIDH), a disabled person is someone who,
because of an impairment, is restricted in performing or cannot
perform an activity in a normal manner. The range of activities in
which a person can be restricted and considered disabled by this
classification is much wider than that used by service providers to
disabled or handicapped people in many parts of the UK and
USA. It is also much wider than the range of activities recommended to local British authorities for identifying disabled people
under the Chronically Sick and Disabled Persons Act of 1970 and
that used in *ad hoc* surveys of disability. The ICIDH does not limit
the losses or abnormalities that characterize impairment, that is
impairment is not contingent upon how the condition developed.
The ICIDH includes ascribed and achieved status, such as genetic
abnormality or the consequences of a road traffic accident.
Moreover, temporary and permanent impairments are included,

and there is no attempt to distinguish between impairments arising from acute conditions or chronic disease.

The questionnaire used to identify disabled adults living in a random sample of households in the London Borough of Lambeth covered most of the categories of disability more comprehensively than ever before. This postal survey estimated that 15 per cent of adults were restricted in one or more areas of their lives because of illness. This percentage is twice the estimate obtained from the OPCS National Survey of disabled people living in the community, partly because the Lambeth study used a wider range of activities to identify disablement, although not the ones specified by ICIDH. While the prevalence of disability increased with age from 7 per cent in the 30–49 age group to 55 per cent among people over 75, each of the age groups, 30–49, 50–64, 65–74, and over 75, contributed almost equal numbers to the total estimate of 30,900 disabled people living in Lambeth. In absolute numbers, disabled people under the age of 65 are as important a segment of the community as are elderly people.

Disabled people aged 25 to 75 who were interviewed after the Lambeth screening survey comprised 28 per cent of the sample who were severely or very severely restricted in their daily activities (arbitrarily defined as an FLP score of 20 or more), a further 27 per cent who were moderately or appreciably restricted (FLP > 8), and 33 per cent with no more than minor disability (FLP < 8). The areas of life in which the disabled respondents were most restricted were recreation and household management. Ambulation came a close second, and the other areas of life, except eating and communication, tied for third place, well below household management and recreation. An image of the typical, physically disabled person as someone severely restricted in self-care activities, reinforced by the definition of disability recommended to local authorities for use in conjunction with the Chronically Sick and Disabled Persons Act, therefore excludes many disabled people significantly restricted in other areas of life. It is equally erroneous to imagine that the majority of disabled people remain static in the severity of their activity restrictions. Over the 2 years of the longitudinal interview study, 70 per cent of the disabled respondents steadily improved, steadily deteriorated, or fluctuated back and forth in their level of disability. Only 30 per cent showed a negligible change in their disability scores.

Efforts to prevent disabilities

Before considering the implications that this alternative view of disabled people has on policy and planning, it is worth reflecting on what has been learned about reducing the level of disability through prevention efforts. Factors such as lowered mortality from infectious and acute illnesses, increased longevity, and survival of those who are impaired have increased the prevalence of persons with disabilities and handicaps associated with impairments and diseases. Prevention of disease through legislative initiatives and lifestyle modification leading to the cessation of smoking, dietary change, regulation of alchohol intake, modification of sexual activity, and safety at home, at work, and on the roads, is likely to assume greater importance in public health policy. Such policy, however, is likely to have little effect on the level of disability or activity restriction in a community such as Lambeth. Chapter 5 showed that the diseases or disorders that contributed most to the level of disability in Lambeth were depression, stroke, arthritis, sciatica, foot trouble, bronchitis, and hypertension. Reduction of cigarette smoking would reduce the incidence of bronchitis, but bronchitis is associated with disability in only one area of life, ambulation. Reducing salt intake may have some part to play in preventing strokes; however, energetic case-finding and treatment of hypertension is likely to have a much greater impact on the prevalence of strokes and hence on disability in the community. With the prospect of many more people in the community being identified as hypertensive than before, it is important to bear in mind that the labelling of some one as hypertensive, without proper explanation and reassurance, and the use of anti-hypertensive drugs can have adverse effects that may themselves be disabling. Because of the large contribution that arthritis and depression make to the amount of disability in the community and because there is as yet no proven effective strategy for preventing these disorders, the primary prevention of disablement is limited.

The high prevalence of unreported and untreated symptoms among disabled people may lead policy-makers and planners to conclude that the screening of disabled people by doctors for unreported and untreated complaints would be a worthwhile investment of time and money, leading to a reduction in disability.

This was thought to be the case in the 1960s, when the finding of unreported medical complaints among the elderly in several surveys led to energetic screening of this section of the community. Not until recently, when randomized controlled trials were carried out, did it become clear that screening alone would not have a major impact on the quality of life of the elderly (Vetter *et al.* 1984). Although there were many symptoms that respondents in the Lambeth survey had not told their doctors about and were not being treated, only three untreated symptoms (constipation, giddiness, and shortness of breath) and four unreported symptoms (spells of feeling hot, nervous, or shaky; diarrhea and/or vomiting; shortness of breath; and giddiness) were associated with disability after accounting for symptoms that had been reported to doctors or were being treated. This finding suggests that the screening for unreported symptoms in disabled people living at home would not have a major effect on the level of disability in Lambeth.

Paradoxically, secondary prevention of disability, if it has anything to do with medical treatment, can be improved, not by treating symptoms more intensively, but by getting general practitioners to review their policies on writing prescriptions for disabled patients. Prescribing drugs was the service that disabled people most frequently sought from their general practitioners and most often received. Analgesics and diuretics were the drugs taken most frequently by disabled people surveyed in Lambeth. Reports of difficulty getting to sleep or staying asleep at night, of frequency or incontinence of urine, of stomach pain occurring between meals, and of constipation, can be due to the adverse effects of diuretics and analgesics. Difficulty getting to sleep or staying asleep at night was associated with restriction in nearly all areas of life. Frequency or incontinence of urine was associated with restriction in body care, ambulation, mobility, rest, recreation and pastime, and social interaction. Constipation and stomach pains were associated with restriction in eating or drinking and recreation and pastime.

These observations suggest that if these symptoms are adverse reactions to drugs, then the level of disability in the community might be reduced by general practitioners prescribing fewer or different medications. This suggestion pre-supposes that general practitioners are aware of both the disabilities and the drugs being taken by their patients. For the most part, general practitioners need to know more about their patients' disabilities so that they can understand fully the potentially adverse effects of prescribing medications. Whether the level of disability would be reduced depends upon the effects of withdrawing or substituting the offending drugs. Routine assessment of functional limitations and activity restrictions in general practice is growing both to identify patients who may be having difficulty functioning without additional services and also to understand more fully the impact of diseases on patients' quality of life (Seltzer *et al* 1984; Patrick and Erickson 1987).

The secondary prevention of disability involves more than the medical treatment of disabling symptoms. Chapter 9 suggested that disabled people with many social contacts were somehow protected from a subsequent decline in their physical and psychosocial functioning, compared with respondents with fewer social contacts, especially in the face of adverse life events. The respondents with few social contacts were unmarried and living alone. The lack of any clear understanding of how social support protects against a decline in functioning and the lack of a proven effective intervention for disabled people with few social contacts, make it difficult to describe the policy and planning implications of the observed relationship between social support and the course of disability.

Respondents with few social contacts were also heavier users of formal services than those with many social contacts. The formal service most frequently used by disabled respondents was the general practitioner. Although disabled people were generally satisfied with the care they were receiving from physicians, dissatisfaction was greater among disabled patients than among those reporting no disability. In particular, respondents who had experienced an adverse life event in the year before their interviews were significantly more likely to be dissatisfied with access to doctors and with their recent medical experiences. Respondents with a higher level of support in completing everyday tasks were less likely to be dissatisfied, in accordance with the view that the lay network plays an important role in how patients view and interact with doctors (Stimson and Webb 1975). Moreover, respondents with higher levels of psychosocial disability, that is, greater restrictions in psychological, social, and mental activity, were significantly and consistently more dissatisfied with their doctors. These respondents expressed doubts about the personal care they were receiving, including length of their medical visits, concern and attention provided by the physician, access to the physician, and other aspects of doctor–patient interactions.

These observations suggest that if disabled respondents with few social contacts are using the general practitioner as a substitute for a lay network, they will be dissatisfied. This supposition would be especially true for people with psychosocial disability who had experienced an adverse life event and who, because of their minimal social contacts, are at risk of steady deterioration in functioning.

It is not surprising that disabled people with few social contacts, especially those with psychosocial disability, would be dissatisfied if they substituted contact with their general practitioners for a large social network. Learning about the psychosocial aspects of disability does not figure highly in the training of physicians. Although more medical schools now provide undergraduates with courses in the social and behavioural sciences, the student alone must integrate such knowledge with the rehabilitation of disabled patients. Even if doctors were properly trained to help people cope with their disabilities, especially in the face of an adverse life event, it is asking a lot for them to provide the kind of support normally provided by a lay network.

The recent growth of self-help groups in Britain and the USA has led some to consider that we are moving towards a society in which people will help each other more. The media regularly include information about specific health organizations, thereby encouraging these groups to expand and meet the needs of people who cannot obtain the support, help, or advice they require from the health or social services. Self-help groups have the potential of allowing disabled people to share their problems with others, to receive technical advice about coping with everyday difficulties, and to deal with stigma. Vachon *et al.* (1980) found that widows assigned to an experimental widow-to-widow programme followed the same general course of adaptation as the control subjects who received no intervention. However, the rate of achieving landmark stages was accelerated for the intervention group, suggesting that such programmes may play an important role in promoting, coping, and increasing people's quality of life.

It is obvious, however, that being a member of a group does not suit everyone. Some people with problems will not participate in groups, purely because they dislike corporate activities or because they feel the group is inappropriate for them. For instance, the group may be too middle-class or too working-class. It is possible that disabled people in the Lambeth survey who had few social contacts, namely the unmarried living alone, would not want to join self-help groups. A few studies have attempted to obtain national data on disabled people who have and have not chosen to join self-help groups. One such study is that of the Parkinson's Disease Society (Oxtoby 1982), which found that meeting with others and companionship was the most appreciated aspect of group activity. However, afflicted people without a spouse were least likely to join the society, and only about a third of the members wanted to take part in branch activities, with 60 per cent of the branch members participating only once or twice in the year before being interviewed.

The observation that the high social contact group in Lambeth contained more employed people than did the low social contact group suggests one way of increasing social contacts for isolated disabled people and perhaps protecting them against a steady deterioration in functioning. In 1978, the Manpower Services Commission in the UK produced a document outlining priorities and policy options to help disabled people find and keep employment. These policies were based on data provided by the Disabled Persons Employment Register. Although more people unable to work because of mental illness and age-related impairments have chosen to register over the past 30 years, the register is still unrepresentative of all disabled people in the community. Perhaps the priorities of the commission need to be reviewed in light of the findings of the Lambeth survey, in which arthritis and depression contributed the most to the overall level of disability. Society may need to shift its priorities from designing schemes to help the severely disabled to encouraging employers to hire and train more people who are less severely disabled, although restricted by depression and arthritis. Programs that increase disabled workers' hopes of finding a job without increasing the chances to find a job may actually be dysfunctional (Frese 1987).

In summary, secondary prevention of disability through screening for untreated medical complaints or by increasing the social networks of disabled people do not appear to be areas that policy-makers and planners can address fruitfully. The former approach is inadvisable because the medical complaints that contribute most to the overall level of disability in the community have already been reported to doctors, and randomized controlled trials have shown that screening alone, for unrecognized health problems, does not have a significant impact on disability. The latter approach is not recommended because we do not know how social support prevents deterioration in functioning or how to increase the social networks of disabled people in a cost-effective way.

Services for disabled people

Our findings confirm that disabled people living in the community are not receiving many of the services for which they are eligible and which might help them to improve their level of functioning or reduce their level of disadvantage. Provision and allocation of services for the disabled is a major priority for policy-makers and planners. A variety of services are available in the UK to promote the social integration of disabled people. Apart from those provided by the National Health Service and by voluntary organizations, an array of supporting services is provided by central and local government sources. Those sources include: the Department of Health and Social Services, which offers artificial limbs, appliances, and mobility schemes; the Department of Employment, which encompasses the Manpower Service Commission's rehabilitation, resettlement, and training services, and the Health and Safety Executive's Employment Medical Advisory Service; local government social services, which offer home adaptations, aids to communication and mobility, home help, chiropody, and recreation; and education and career services.

Respondents in the Lambeth survey were asked about their use of health and social services. Although disabled respondents were heavy users of general practitioners, out-patient clinics, and casualty departments, they encountered other health professionals and used personal social services less frequently. Seventy per cent of the disabled had never seen a chiropodist; 18 per cent had never seen an optician; and 29 per cent had never seen a dentist. The number of disabled people receiving domiciliary services was also small. In the 2 weeks prior to the survey interview, the service most received was a home help (89 per cent), followed by meals-on-wheels (30 per cent), social worker (27 per cent), district nurse (25 per cent), and physiotherapist (19 per cent). Even allowing for the wide range of severity of disability in the sample, the low use of formal services (other than the general practitioner) might lead people who believe in an equal distribution of the same type of resources among disabled with similar needs, to conclude that the disabled residents in Lambeth were not receiving all the services that might help them.

It is well-known that general practitioners have more contact with physically disabled people than any other professional or agency. Harris (1971) found that 90 per cent of registered disabled people had consulted a physician at least once over a 12-month period. Moreover, the Consumers Association (1978) found that the general practitioner was the only person with whom one in 10 disabled people had any contact. Because general practitioners see more of disabled people than any other professional, they are in the best position to refer patients to other caring agencies such as the social services (Seebohm Report 1968).

In contrast to the use of personal social services, 31 per cent of the disabled people in Lambeth had contacted a general practitioner within the 2 weeks before being interviewed. The doctor referred these patients to other formal services (except the hospital) or ordered appliances or aids for them relatively infrequently. Another study has found that general practitioners know about only 60 per cent of the difficulties with daily living reported by their disabled patients and even less about the aids, appliances, and services they use (Patrick *et al.* 1982). These sorts of observations suggest that general practitioners are responsible, in part, for disabled people not receiving all the services that could help them (*British Medical Journal* 1979).

These observations do not take into account, however, that referring disabled people to the social services or other agencies is a way of rationing limited resources to those most in need (see Chapter 7). The general practitioner is involved in at least three steps: professional assessment, decision on whether to treat or turn away, and decision on whether to treat at the initial doctor–patient contact or to move the patient further into the provision system. The general practitioner acts as a gatekeeper to the other formal services, primarily rationing services to those most in need.

The FLP gives a measure of an individual's perceived dysfunction in the main areas of life, but, as explained in Chapter 7, an overall or category score on the FLP is too non-specific to use as a proxy for professional judgment of normative need for services. Individual statements on the FLP provide a better, though by no means perfect, proxy for normative need of aids to alleviate limitations. Within this survey population there was relatively little unmet need, whereby the respondent reported a functional limitation but did not have any aids to help with it. The ambulation severity scores indicated, however, that it was the less severely disabled who reported having limitations and no aids. The extent of unacceptably met need was very low for all categories, whereas acceptably met need was high. Unperceived need, whereby a functional limitation was expressed without the possession or need for aids, occurred in many categories especially for limitations in putting on socks, shoes, and stockings, dressing, difficulty moving in and out of bed and bath, and walking and using stairs. Very few respondents had any needs that were met only partially. At the same time surprisingly few respondents who had aids did not want anymore.

The frequent occurrence of unperceived need might mean that some disabled people do not know how aids can help them or do not recognize their eligibility for aids. However, a person with a functional limitation who does not possess or express a need for an aid may not want one. Although fear of stigma or feeling demeaned are possible explanations, it is more likely that disabled people simply have a better idea of what aids will benefit them in their particular circumstances than a researcher or professional.

Increasing cash benefits for disabled people

It has been suggested that policy-makers and planners should consider ways of getting services to more disabled people (*British Medical Journal* 1979). Methods proposed include: involving general practitioners in locating disabled people, providing primary care teams with a contact person in social service departments, distributing reply-paid cards to all households to enquire about their health status, poviding written information on services available for households, and setting up telephone advisory services. The Lambeth survey found little comparative need for aids, and where this need did exist, it was among the less severely disabled. Findings from this survey, therefore, do not support an 'all-out effort' to get more services to more disabled people. Resources are limited and what resources there are appear to be going to those with the greatest comparative need. Bypassing the general practitioner and primary rationing in the face of limited resources will only bring secondary and tertiary rationing mechanisms into play. If more disabled people are fed into the provision system without a corresponding increase in resources, then waiting lists for services will lengthen (secondary rationing) or the quantity and quality of the services given to individual clients will be reduced (tertiary rationing). If services are diluted too much, then the benefit of extending services to more people may be weakened.

Although disabled people may not demand services, it does not mean that they do not want help of any sort. Chapter 10 describes the wide variety of ways in which disabled people change their lifestyles to cope with disadvantage. The way disabled people choose to cope with disadvantage, however, does not always ensure that they remain integrated in society. For example, three distinct mechanisms were described for coping with work handicaps: accepting help from colleagues and employers, changing jobs, and accepting unemployment. Two out of these three strategies led to the segregation of the respondent from the mainstream of society. One respondent needed help in getting access to social clubs for able-bodied people. The other needed her employer to give the work she could not cope with to other people, or to be able to share her work with a part-time, able-bodied secretary. A large number of possible improvements exist to aid the increased integration of disabled people in society. However, devising and providing services to meet every need of handicapped people, many of which are probably specific and possibly unique, is neither practically nor economically feasible. The only viable option is to make compensatory provision for handicap in cash, allowing disabled people to buy what they need. Clearly stringent criteria of eligibility will be required to implement such a policy.

Cash provision alone would not be sufficient to reduce the prevalence and degree of handicap or disadvantage in the community. Cash would enable disabled people to purchase services they believe would overcome the main and individualistic barriers that create unequal opportunities and participation. But society must be willing and able to receive these people, that is willing to care for the needs of strangers (Churchill 1987). Disabled people and other disadvantaged groups must be taken into account by policy-making and planning at all levels and in all areas of life. Instead of thinking in terms of disabled and non-disabled populations, planners and policy-makers need to think in terms of one population or one community, a significant proportion of which will have a diversity of activity restrictions and/or handicaps. Society's attitudes are beginning to move in this direction primarily through media education and increasing exposure to disabled people in everyday life. There is growing experience of disabled people who, with appropriate supports, lead full and independent lives. Such attitudes, however, must be reinforced by legislation.

In the USA, national provision for disabled people has followed the enactment of federal disability laws passed by Congress over the last few decades. These laws mark a shift in US public policy, from a focus on the provision of personal services for disabled individuals to one that concentrates more on providing cash benefits and that encourages equality or established protection and advocacy systems for disabled people. Much of the US legislation is aimed at making the environment accessible to all citizens (De Jong and Lifchez 1983). The two largest federal income-transfer programmes for disabled people—Social Security Disability Insurance and Supplemental Security Income—have more than doubled in cash payments over the last 20 years. Much responsibility for provision for disabled people is also shifting to the States. Thus, attempts to enhance the quality of life for disabled Americans are primarily legislative initiatives for the protection of civil rights, which are intended to promote social integration and to reduce disadvantage.

Like most public policy shifts, however, increasing the provision of cash benefits to disabled people may also have unintended consequences. Disability income maintenance can confirm an individual's devalued, disabled, and patient status. Compensation can enhance withdrawal from interaction with others such as work associates and thereby sustain an isolated, stigmatized existence. As Charmaz (1983) describes eloquently, 'chronically ill persons frequently experience a crumbling away of their former self-images without simultaneous development of equally valued new ones'. To avoid these conflicting consequences, income maintenance must be accompanied by national legislation and social services that help disabled people participate in meaningful social activity that is valued by all in the community.

The Lambeth disablement studies do not support a policy of screening for untreated symptoms or of artificially substituting informal support for a deficient social network as a means of secondarily preventing disability. A time-consuming and costly policy aimed at increasing the amount of personal social services for disabled people does not seem to be a high priority, especially at a time of increased resources rationing. The reduction of handicap and the promotion of equal opportunity and participation of disabled people are the goals with which policy-makers and planners should concern themselves. Further research on disablement should investigate methods of determining eligibility for a handicap allowance and gain a greater understanding of handicap in order to enumerate the key policies needed to reduce disadvantage.

References

British Medical Journal (1979). Are they being served? *British Medical Journal* **1**, 147–8.

Charmaz, K. (1983). Loss of self: a fundamental form of suffering in the chronically ill. *Sociology of Health and Illness* **5**, 168–95.

Churchill, L. R. (1987). *Rationing health care in America: perceptions and principles of justice.* University of Notre Dame Press, Notre Dame, USA.

Consumers Association (1978). *Managing at home.* A Which Campaign Report. Consumers Association, London.

DeJong, G. and Lifchez, R. (1983). Physical disability and public policy. *Scientific American* **248**, 40–48.

Frese, M. (1987). Alleviating depression in the unemployed: adequate financial support, hope and early retirement. *Social Science and Medicine* **25**, 213–15.

Harris, A. I. (1971). *Handicapped and impaired in Great Britain.* HMSO, London.

Manpower Services Commission (1978). *Developing employment and training services for disabled people: an MSC programme.* Manpower Services Commission, London.

Oxtoby, M. (1982). *Parkinson's disease patients and their special needs.* Parkinson's Disease Society, London.

Patrick, D. L. and Erickson, P. (1987). Assessing health-related quality of life for clinical decision making. In *Quality of life: assessment and application.* (eds S. R. Walker and R. M. Rosser) MTP Press Limited, Lancaster.

Patrick, D. L., Peach, H., and Gregg, I. (1982). Disablement and care: a comparison of patient views and general practitioner knowledge. *Journal of the Royal College of General Practitioners* **32**, 429–34.

Seebohm Report (1968). Report of the Committee on Local Authority and Allied Personal Social Services. HMSO, London.

Seltzer, G. B., Granger, C. V., Wineberg, D. E., *et al.* (1984). Functional assessment in primary care. In *Functional assessment in rehabilitation medicine.* (eds C. V. Granger and G. E. Gresham). pp. 289–305, Williams & Wilkins, Baltimore.

Stimson, G. and Webb, B. (1975). *Going to see the doctor: the consultation process in general practice.* Routledge and Kegan Paul, London.

Vachon, M., Lyall, W., Rodgers, J., Freedman-Letofsky, K., and Freeman, S. (1980). A controlled study of self-help for widows. *American Journal of Psychiatry* **137**, 1380–4.

Vetter, N. J., Jones, D. A., and Victor, C. R. (1984). Effect of health visitors working with elderly patients in general practice: a randomized controlled trial. *British Medical Journal* **288**, 369–72.

Appendix 1.

Lambeth disability screening questionnaire

LAMBETH HEALTH SURVEY

The following questions apply to EVERYONE AGED 16 OR OVER living in this household. Please answer every question as well as you can, as shown in the examples below.

EXAMPLE 1 *(for when someone has difficulty)*

WHO has difficulty with any of the following?	The first names and ages of everyone having this difficulty are	No-one
Getting around the house without help		

EXAMPLE 2 *(for when no-one has difficulty)*

WHO has difficulty with any of the following?	The first names and ages of everyone having this difficulty are	No-one
Getting around the house without help		

START HERE

1. WHO has difficulty with any of the following?	The first names and ages of everyone having this difficulty are	No-one
a. Walking without help		
b. Getting outside the house without help		
c. Crossing the road without help		
d. Travelling on a bus or train without help		

1   *Please continue on the back of this page*

2. WHO has difficulty with any of the following?	The first names and ages of everyone having this difficulty are	No-one
a. Getting in and out of bed or chair without help		
b. Dressing or undressing without help		
c. Kneeling or bending over without help		
d. Going up or down stairs without help		
e. Having a bath or all over wash without help		
f. Holding or gripping (for example a comb or a pen) without help		
g. Getting to and using the toilet without help		

3. WHO has any of the following problems?	The first names and ages of everyone having this difficulty are	No-one
a. Difficulty with spells of giddiness or fits		
b. Frequent falls		
c. Weakness or paralysis of arms or legs		
d. A stroke		
e. Difficulty seeing newspaper print even with glasses		
f. Difficulty recognizing people across the road even with glasses		
g. Hearing difficulties		
h. Loss of whole or *significant part* of an arm, hand, leg or foot		
i. Controlling bowels or bladder		

2

Please continue on next page

4. WHO is limited in doing any of the following BECAUSE OF ILLNESS OR DISABILITY?

	The first names and ages of everyone having this difficulty are	No-one
a. Working at all		
b. Doing the job of their choice		
c. Doing housework		
d. Visiting family or friends		

5. *If you have written ANY names in Questions 1-4,* please tell us what their major illness or disability is?

First names and ages of anyone mentioned in Questions 1-4	Please describe their major illness or disability below

6. Does *anyone else* in your household have an illness or disability which affects their activities in any way?

First names and ages of anyone with illness or disability	What is the major illness or disability?	Please describe activity (e.g. playing sports, sewing, going to the pub)

3   *Please continue on the back of this page*

ALL INFORMATION CONFIDENTIAL

Please complete below EVEN IF NO-ONE IS ILL OR DISABLED. We need this information to plan services for
EVERYONE in Lambeth.

List Below EVERYONE, INCLUDING YOURSELF, living in this household.
Give the full name together with details for EVERYONE

1-5

6	NAME Write below Surname – Forename(s)	7 SEX Tick box Male Female (1) (2)		8-11 YEAR OF BIRTH Write Below	MARITAL STATUS Write below—Single, Married, Widowed, Divorced or Separated	12	13 CURRENTLY EMPLOYED? Tick box Yes(1) No(2)		14
0									
1									
2									
3									
4									
5									
6									
7									
8									
9									

15   16-18   19   20-21   22-27   80

SINCE WORK CAN AFFECT HEALTH, PLEASE COMPLETE FOR THE HEAD OF YOUR HOUSEHOLD ONLY
(Person with responsibility for supporting household or for rent/accommodation).

First Name and Age of HEAD OF HOUSEHOLD	What job does he/she do? (If Head is retired, unemployed, or not present, what was the job he/she held for most of his/her working life?)

Is (or was) the Head of the Household	☐ a manager working for an employer?	☐ a foreman or super- visor working for an employer?	☐ working for an employer?	☐ self-employed?
What qualifications, if any, were needed to obtain this job?				
What does the firm or organization do or make?				

Signature of person filling in form

WE APPRECIATE YOUR CO-OPERATION. THANK YOU.
Please check carefully that ALL questions on every page are answered.

4

Appendix 2.
Functional limitations profile

This document describes the use of the Functional Limitations Profile (FLP), a British Version of the Sickness Impact Profile, translated into British English and rescored using British item weights.

For additional information contact:

Dr. Donald Patrick,

Department of Health Services, SC–37,

School of Public Health and Community Medicine,

University of Washington,

Seattle, Washington 98195.

Telephone: (206) 543–8866

This Appendix contains interview instructions, scoring instructions, and FLP items.

The following instructions are for the **Interviewer-administered questionnaire**

Interview Instructions

SAY TO ALL VERBATIM

I want to talk to you about the things you normally do every day.

I am going to read out some statements which describe things people often do when they are not well. Even if you think you are well, some of these statements may stand out, because they describe you and are related to your health. Listen to each statement, think of yourself *today* and tell me if it describes you or not. For example, I might read the statement, 'I am not driving my car'. If you agree with this statement, you should tell me (agree/disagree is the best response pattern). I will then ask, 'Is this due to you health?' Please answer 'yes' or 'no'. If you have not been driving for some time due to your health and are still not driving today, you should respond 'agree'.

(HOSPITAL) If you are in hospital today, you are here because of your state of health, and you are not doing a number of the things you usually do. For instance, if driving is usual for you, then you are *not* driving today because you are in hospital, and you should agree with this statement.

If you never drive or are not driving today because your car is being repaired, you should not respond that the statement is due to your health. Ask me to repeat a statement or slow down if you do not understand. Remember we are interested in both recent or longstanding changes in your health.

The following instructions are for the **Self-administered questionnaire:**

Introduction to the respondent

We are interested in the activities that you do in carrying on your life and any changes that describe you today that are related to your health.

This booklet lists statements that describe things people often do when they are not well. Even if you think you are well, some of these statements may stand out, because they describe you and are related to your health. As you read each statement in the questionnaire, think of yourself today. When you read a statement that describes you and is related to your health, place a tick on the line to the right of the statement. For example:

I am not driving my car   _____

If you have not been driving for some time because of your health and are still not driving today, you should tick this statement. On the other hand, if you never drive or are not driving today because your car is being repaired, you should *not* tick it. Tick a statement *only* if you are *sure* it describes you and is due to health.

NOTE: At the bottom of each page of the self-administered questionnaire, you may wish to ask the respondent to indicate that he or she has read all statements on the page by ticking the following statement:

TICK HERE WHEN YOU HAVE READ ALL STATEMENTS ON THIS PAGE   _____

Answering queries that may arise

'*I've never been able to do that.*' **Say**: Yes, we do want to know about things you have never been able to do.

'*I've not been able to do that for some time.*' **Say**: We want to know about all recent or long-standing changes in the things you do.

'*Some days I can do that, some days I can't.*' **Say**: Think of yourself *today*.

'*It's due to my age.*' **Say**: Would you say that was due to your *health* or not?

'*None of this applies to me; I'm perfectly healthy.*' **Say**: A few of the statements may apply to you. It is therefore important that we do check them all, since we are comparing healthy people with less healthy people.

Additional queries:

Scoring instructions

There are 12 category scores, 2 dimension scores, and an overall FLP score.

Category scores

The percentage score is calculated for each category by adding the scale values for each item with which the respondent agrees and considers due to his/her health (or ticked items) and dividing by the maximum possible dysfunction score for the FLP. This figure is then multiplied by 100 to obtain the FLP category score.

Dimension scores

Two dimension scores may be calculated. The *physical* dimension score is obtained by adding the scale values for each item with which the respondent agrees and considers due to his/her health (or ticked items) with the categories of ambulation, body care and movement, mobility, and household management, dividing by the maximum possible dysfunction score for these categories (4345), and then mulltiplying by 100. The *psychosocial* dimension score is obtained by adding the scale values for each item ticked within recreation and pastime, social interaction, emotion, alertness, and sleep and rest, dividing by the maximum possible dysfunction sore for these categories (3667), and then multiplying by 100. The scores for the remaining categories are always calculated individually.

Overall FLP score

The overall score for the FLP is calculated by adding the scale values for each item with which the respondent agrees and considers to be due to his/her health (or ticked items) across all 12 categories and dividing by the maximum possible dysfunction score for the FLP (9923). This figure is then multiplied by 100 to obtain the FLP overall score.

Each item within the 12 categories is listed on the following pages along with the scale values coded to one decimal as follows:

1. Only items with which the respondent agrees and considers due to his/her health (or ticked items) should be included in the calculation of FLP category, dimension, and overall score.
2. Following each item is the scale value or weight for that item (e.g., item 1 has a scale value of 5.4).
3. The maximum possible scale value is shown following the title of each category (e.g., the ambulation category has a maximum possible score of 100.6.
4. The maximum possible score for the physical dimension is 434.5 while the maximum possible score for the psychosocial dimension is 366.7.
5. The maximum possible score for the FLP is 992.3 which is the denomintor for calculating the percent score for the entire FLP.

6. A special case of category and FLP overall score concerns the work category. Item 128 has a weight of 361 indicating an unusually high scale value. The scale value for this item has been statistically adjusted to take into account the fact that when item 128 is ticked no other item in the work category can be ticked. Please note that the maximum possible score for the work category is not the sum of the individual items, but is instead 70% of the total. This value was determined using the distribution of scores on the work category.

Also, with respect to the work category there are two special considerations in scoring:

1. When a respondent agrees with either,
   (a) 'If you are retired, was your retirement due to your health?' or
   (b) 'If you are not retired, but are *not* working, is this due to your health?'
   he or she is instructed to skip category W—Work. In scoring the questionnaire for respondents who answer *Yes* to either of these questions, *item 128* should be ticked.

Ambulation items (maximum possible score = 1006)

The following statements describe walking and use of stairs. Remember, think of yourself today. *If 'AGREE', PROBE*: Is this due to your health?

1. I walk shorter distances or often stop for a rest. – (054)
2. I do not walk up or down hills. – (064)
3. I only use stairs with a physical aid; for example, a handrail, stick, or crutches. – (082)
4. I only go up and down stairs with assistance from someone else. – (087)
5. I get about in a wheelchair. – (121)
6. I do not walk at all. – (126)
7. I walk by myself but with some difficulty; for example, I limp, wobble, stumble, or I have a stiff leg. – (071)
8. I only walk with help from someone else. – (098)
9. I go up and down stairs more slowly; for example, one step at a time or I often have to stop. – (062)
10. I do not use stairs at all. – (106)
11. I get about only by using a walking frame, crutches, stick, walls, or hold onto furniture. – (096)
12. I walk more slowly. – (039)

TICK HERE WHEN YOU HAVE READ ALL
STATEMENTS ON THIS PAGE   —

Body care and movement items (maximum possible score = 1927)

The following statements describe how you move about, bath, go to the toilet, dress yourself today. *If 'AGREE', PROBE*: Is this due to your health?

13. I make difficult movements with help; for example, getting in or out of the bath or a car. – (082)
14. I do not get in and out of bed or chairs without the help of a person or mechanical aid. – (100)
15. I only stand for short periods of time. – (067)
16. I do not keep my balance. – (093)
17. I move my hands or fingers with some difficulty or limitation. – (066)
18. I only stand up with someone's help. – (093)
19. I kneel, stoop or bend down only by holding onto something. – (061)
20. I am in a restricted position all the time. – (124)
21. I am very clumsy. – (047)
22. I get in and out of bed or chairs by grasping something for support or by using a stick or walking frame. – (079)
23. I stay lying down most of the time. – (120)
24. I change position frequently. – (0513)
25. I hold onto something to move myself around in bed. – (082)
26. I do not bathe myself completely; for example, I need help with bathing. – (085)
27. I do not bathe myself at all, but am bathed by someone else. – (100)
28. I use a bedpan with help. – (107)
29. I have trouble putting on my shoes, socks, or stockings. – (054)
30. I do not have control of my bladder. – (122)
31. I do not fasten my clothing; for example, I require assistance with buttons, zips, or shoelaces. – (068)
32. I spend most of the time partly dressed or in pyjamas. – (075)
33. I do not have control of my bowels. – (124)
34. I dress myself, but do so very slowly. – (043)
35. I only get dressed with someone's help. – (082)

TICK HERE WHEN YOU HAVE READ ALL
STATEMENTS ON THIS PAGE   –

Mobility items (maximum posible score = 0727)

These next statements describe how you get about the house and outside. *If 'AGREE' PROBE*: Is this due to your health?

36. I only get about in one building. — (076)
37. I stay in one room. — (101)
38. I stay in bed more. — (091)
39. I stay in bed most of the time. — (114)
40. I do not use public transport now. — (052)
41. I stay at home most of the time. — (079)
42. I only go out if there is a lavatory nearby. — (064)
43. I do not go into town. — (047)
44. I only stay away from home for short periods. — (046)
45. I do not get about in the dark or in places that are not lit unless I have someone to help. — (057)

TICK HERE WHEN YOU HAVE READ ALL
STATEMENTS ON THIS PAGE —

Household management items (maximum possible socre = 0685)

The following statements describe your daily work, around the home. When you answer, think of yourself today *If 'AGREE' PROBE*: Is this due to your health?

46. I only do housework or work around the house for short periods of time or I rest often. — (050)
47. I do less of the daily household chores than I would usually do. — (037)
48. I do not do any of the daily household chores that I would usually do. — (090)
49. I do not do any of the maintenance or repair work that I would usually do in my home or garden. — (075)
50. I do not do any of the shopping that I would usually do. — (084)
51. I do not do any of the cleaning that I would usually do. — (078)
52. I have difficulty using my hands; for example, turning taps, using kitchen gadgets, sewing, or doing repairs. — (078)
53. I do not do any of the clothes washing that I would usually do. — (075)
54. I do not do heavy work around the house. — (059)

55. I have given up taking care of personal or household business affairs; for example, paying bills, banking, or doing household accounts. — (069)

TICK HERE WHEN YOU HAVE READ ALL STATEMENTS ON THIS PAGE —

(**Maximum possible physical dimension score** = 4345)

Recreation and pastime items (maximum possible score = 0383)

The following statements describe the activities you usually do in your spare time, for relaxation, entertainment or just to pass the time. Again think of yourself today. *If 'AGREE' PROBE*: Is this due to your health?

56. I spend shorter periods of time on my hobbies and recreation. — (032)
57. I go out less often to enjoy myself. — (027)
58. I am cutting down on some of my usual inactive pastimes; for example, I watch TV less, play cards less, or read less. — (050)
59. I am not doing any of my usual inactive pastimes; for example, I do not watch TV, play cards, or read. — (091)
60. I am doing more inactive pastimes instead of my other usual activities. — (043)
61. I take part in fewer community activities. — (025)
62. I am cutting down on some of my usual physical recreation or more active pastimes. — (034)
63. I am not doing any of my usual physical recreation or more active pastimes. — (081)

TICK HERE WHEN YOU HAVE READ ALL STATEMENTS ON THIS PAGE —

Social interaction items (maximum possible score = 1289)

These statements describe your contact with family and friends today. *If 'AGREE' PROBE*: Is this due to your health?

64. I go out less often to visit people. — (031)
65. I do not go out at all to visit people. — (091)
66. I show less interest in other people's problems; for example, I don't listen when they tell me about their problems, I don't offer to help. — (050)

67. I am often irritable with those around me; for example, I snap at people or criticize easily. — (064)
68. I show less affection. — (044)
69. I take part in fewer social activities than I used to; for example, I go to fewer parties or social events. — (025)
70. I am cutting down the length of visits with friends. — (031)
71. I avoid having visitors. — (073)
72. My sexual activity is decreased. — (064)
73. I often express concern over what might be happening to my health. — (044)
74. I talk less with other people. — (044)
75. I make many demands on other people; for example, I insist that they do things for me or tell them how to do things. — (076)
76. I stay alone much of the time. — (091)
77. I am disagreeable with my family; for example, I act spitefully or stubbornly. — (086)
78. I frequently get angry with my family; for example, I hit them, scream, or throw things at them. — (103)
79. I isolate myself as much as I can from the rest of my family. — (100)
80. I pay less attention to the children. — (059)
81. I refuse contact with my family; for example, I turn away from them. — (109)
82. I do not look after my children or family as well as I usually do. — (066)
83. I do not joke with members of my family as much as I usually do. — (038)

TICK HERE WHEN YOU HAVE READ ALL
STATEMENTS ON THIS PAGE —

Emotion items (maximum possible score = 0693)

The next statements describe your feelings and behavior. Again think of yourself today. *If 'AGREE' PROBE*: Is this due to your health?

84. I say how bad or useless I am; for example, that I am a burden on others. — (089)
85. I laugh or cry suddenly. — (058)
86. I often moan and groan because of pain or discomfort. — (067)
87. I have attempted suicide. — (141)
88. I behave nervously or restlessly. — (048)
89. I keep rubbing or holding areas of my body that hurt or are uncomfortable. — (059)

90. I am irritable and impatient with myself; for example, I run myself down, I swear at myself, I blame myself for things that happen. — (079)
91. I talk hopelessly about the future. — (096)
92. I get sudden frights. — (056)

TICK HERE WHEN YOU HAVE READ ALL STATEMENTS ON THIS PAGE —

Alertness items (maximum possible score = 0711)

93. I am confused and start to do more than one thing at a time. — (074)
94. I have more minor accidents for example; I drop things, I trip and fall, I bump into things. — (090)
95. I react slowly to things that are said or done. — (052)
96. I do not finish things I start. — (045)
97. I have difficulty reasoning and solving problems; for example, making plans, making decisions, learning new things. — (078)
98. I sometimes get confused; for example, I do not know where I am, who is around, or what day it is. — (115)
99. I forget a lot; for example, things that happened recently, where I put things, or to keep appointments. — (085)
100. I do not keep my attention on any activity for long. — (052)
101. I make more mistakes than usual. — (049)
102. I have difficulty doing things which involve thought and concentration. — (071)

TICK HERE WHEN YOU HAVE READ ALL STATEMENTS ON THIS PAGE —

Sleep and rest items (maximum possible score = 0591)

These statements describe your sleep and rest activities today. *If 'AGREE' PROBE*: Is this due to your health?

103. I spend much of the day lying down to rest. — (096)
104. I sit for much of the day. — (062)
105. I sleep or doze most of the time, day and night. — (111)
106. I lie down to rest more often during the day. — (072)
107. I sit around half asleep. — (084)

108. I sleep less at night; for example, I wake up easily, I
     don't fall asleep for a long time, or I keep waking up. — (086)
109. I sleep or doze more during the day.   — (080)
TICK HERE WHEN YOU HAVE READ ALL
STATEMENTS ON THIS PAGE   —
(**Maximum possible psychosocial dimension score** = 3667)

Eating items (maximum possible score = 0706)

The following statements describe your eating and drinking habits. *If
'AGREE' PROBE:* Is this due to your health?

110. I eat much less than usual.   — (034)
111. I feed myself but only with specially prepared food or
     special utensils.   — (076)
112. I eat special or different food; for example, I follow a
     soft food, bland, low salt, low fat, or low sugar diet. — (052)
113. I eat no food at all, but I take liquids.   — (113)
114. I just pick or nibble at my food.   — (039)
115. I drink less fluids.   — (033)
116. I feed myself with help from someone else.   — (095)
117. I do not feed myself at all, but have to be fed.   — (121)
Interviewer may code
118. I eat no food at all except by tubes or intravenous
     infusion.   — (143)
TICK HERE WHEN YOU HAVE READ ALL
STATEMENTS ON THIS PAGE   —

Communication items (maximum possible score = 0685)

I am going to read out some statements about how much you talk to other
people and write. Please think about yourself today. *If 'AGREE'
PROBE*: Is this due to your health?

119. I have trouble writing or typing.   — (050)
120. I communicate mostly by nodding my head, pointing,
     or using sign language, or other gestures.   — (127)
121. My speech is understood only by a few people who
     know me well.   — (094)
122. I often lose control of my voice when I talk; for
     example, my voice gets louder or softer, or changes
     unexpectedly.   — (059)
123. I don't write except to sign my name.   — (084)

124. I carry on a conversation only when very close to
     other people or looking directly at them. — (059)
125. I speak with difficulty; for example, I get stuck for
     words, I stutter, I stammer, I slur my words. — (076)
126. I am understood with difficulty. — (089)
127. I do not speak clearly when I am under stress. — (047)
TICK HERE WHEN YOU HAVE READ ALL
STATEMENTS ON THIS PAGE —

Work items (maximum possible score = 0520)

I am going to read out some statements about work. As I read them out
think of yourself today. If today is not a working day for you, think about
your last working day. *If 'AGREE' PROBE*: Is this due to your health?

Self-administered: The next group of statements has to do with any
work you usually do other than managing your home. By this we mean
anything that you regard as work that you do on a regular basis.

Do you usually do work other than managing your home? Yes No
If yes, complete the work section.
If no:
Are you retired? Yes No
If you are retired, was your retirement due to your health? Yes No
If you are not retired, but are not working, is this due
to your health? Yes No

If yes, please tick item 128 and skip the rest of the items in this section
If no, please skip this section

128. I do not work at all.
     (includes retired because of health) — (361)
129. I do part of my job at home. — (040)
130. I am not getting as much work done as usual. — (041)
131. I often get irritable with my workmates; for example,
     I snap at them or criticize them easily. — (042)
132. I work shorter hours. — (052)
133. I only do light work. — (056)
134. I only work for short periods of time or often stop to
     rest. — (065)
135. I work at my usual job but with some changes; for
     example, I use different tools or special aids, or I
     swap jobs with someone else. — (036)
136. I do not do my job as carefully and accurately as
     usual. — (050)
(**Maximum possible FLP score** = 9923)

Index